S.I.T Workout Quick 7 Minute Home Workout

Maxim Feldhinkel

Published by Maxim Feldhinkel, 2025.

S.I.T Workout: Quick 7 Minute Home Workout

First edition. January 19, 2025.

Written by Maxim Feldhinkel.

Table of contents:

Introduction:

Here you will begin your path to a better, fitter self! Finding the time to exercise in today's hectic lifestyle might seem like an insurmountable obstacle. Making time for fitness a priority between job, family, social obligations, and everything else may be challenging. But what if you didn't need hours at the gym to stay in shape? What if just seven minutes could make a noticeable difference in your fitness?

This is where the 7-minute S.I.T. workout comes in. S.I.T. – which stands for **Short Intense Training** – is a revolutionary workout method designed to give you maximum results in minimal time. No matter your schedule—whether you're a parent, a working professional, or just trying to get in a little exercise here and there, this workout provides an efficient solution for building strength, improving endurance, and boosting overall fitness.

Here, you'll find comprehensive information on how to make the S.I.T. workout a regular part of your routine. If you want to learn how to incorporate exercise into your everyday life but don't know where to start, this book will walk you through the science, benefits, and the process of creating your own workout regimen.

If you follow this plan to the letter, you will be well-equipped to start your own 7-minute S.I.T. exercise and get its advantages. Get ready to start your journey to a healthier, more energised, and stronger version of yourself by taking a deep breath. The adventure is about to start.

Chapter 1: What is S.I.T.?

In the world of fitness, time has become one of the most significant barriers to consistent exercise. Finding the time to exercise effectively might seem like an insurmountable obstacle when you consider everyone's hectic schedules, job obligations, and personal duties. Enter Sprint-Interval Training, or S.I.T., a groundbreaking fitness method designed to maximize results in minimal time.

S.I.T. has gained immense popularity due to its simplicity, accessibility, and unparalleled efficiency. But what exactly is S.I.T., and why has it become a go-to strategy for fitness enthusiasts and beginners alike? This chapter will explore the fundamentals of S.I.T., its principles, and its unique advantages over traditional training methods.

Definition of S.I.T.

Quick, all-out bursts of effort (sprints) are interspersed with longer, less strenuous recovery intervals in sprint-interval training, a high-intensity workout approach. Unlike steady-state cardio, where you maintain a consistent pace over an extended duration, S.I.T. pushes your body to its limits for brief moments, creating a "shock" effect on your cardiovascular system, muscles, and metabolism.

The essence of S.I.T. lies in its efficiency: by performing short, explosive intervals, you can achieve results comparable to—or even better than—traditional workouts that require significantly more time.

For example, a S.I.T. session might involve 20 seconds of maximum-effort sprinting followed by 40 seconds of slow jogging or walking. This pattern is repeated multiple times, creating a workout that is both time-effective and highly intense.

How S.I.T. works: The science behind the method

S.I.T. operates on a principle called **metabolic overload**. When you perform an exercise at maximum intensity, your body consumes a significant amount of energy in a short period. This intense energy demand creates a cascade of physiological responses:

> **1.Oxygen debt**: During the high-intensity sprint phase, your body relies on anaerobic energy systems because oxygen delivery cannot keep up with the demand. This leads to oxygen debt, which your body must repay during the recovery phase and after the workout, a process known as **excess post-exercise oxygen consumption (EPOC)**.

> **2.Increased heart rate and cardiovascular strain**: The rapid bursts of effort cause your heart rate to spike, improving cardiovascular efficiency over time. Your heart becomes stronger, and your body becomes better at pumping blood and delivering oxygen to working muscles.

3.Muscle fiber activation: S.I.T. recruits fast-twitch muscle fibers, which are responsible for explosive movements. These fibers are often underutilized during steady-state cardio, making S.I.T. an excellent way to build strength and power.

4.Hormonal boost: Intense exercise stimulates the release of key hormones such as adrenaline, noradrenaline, and growth hormone. These hormones enhance fat burning, improve energy levels, and support muscle recovery.

5.Improved Insulin sensitivity: Research shows that S.I.T. can improve the body's ability to regulate blood sugar, making it an effective tool for preventing or managing conditions like type 2 diabetes.

The key features of S.I.T.

S.I.T. distinguishes itself through several unique characteristics:

1.Intensity over duration: S.I.T. prioritizes quality over quantity. Workouts are brief but highly challenging, pushing your body to its limits in a short timeframe.

2.No equipment needed: Many S.I.T. workouts rely on bodyweight exercises or activities like running, jumping, or cycling. This makes it accessible to anyone, regardless of fitness level or gym access.

3.Adaptability: S.I.T. can be customized to suit various fitness levels, goals, and preferences. Whether you're a beginner or a seasoned athlete, you can modify the duration and intensity of sprints and recovery phases.

4.Versatility: S.I.T. is not limited to sprinting alone. It can be applied to a variety of exercises, including jumping jacks, burpees, squats, or even swimming.

5.Time-efficient: The cornerstone of S.I.T. is its ability to deliver results in as little as 7–15 minutes.

S.I.T. vs. Traditional training methods

To truly understand S.I.T., it's important to compare it with other common workout approaches:

1.S.I.T.   vs.   Steady-state   cardio
Steady-state cardio involves maintaining a moderate, consistent pace (e.g., jogging or cycling) for an extended period. While effective for improving endurance, it requires more time and does not provide the same metabolic benefits as S.I.T. **Key Difference**: S.I.T. burns more calories in less time, boosts metabolism for hours after the workout, and activates fast-twitch muscle fibers often overlooked in steady-state cardio.

2.S.I.T.   vs.   HIIT   (High-Intensity   Interval   Training)
Although similar, S.I.T. is a more intense subset of HIIT. While HIIT incorporates a mix of high and moderate intensities, S.I.T. focuses solely on maximum effort during the work

phases.

Key difference: S.I.T. is shorter and more intense, making it ideal for those who want to push their limits in a very brief session.

Benefits of S.I.T.

The appeal of S.I.T. is in the many ways in which it improves health and wellness:

1.Improved cardiovascular health: By improving oxygen supply and strengthening the heart, regular S.I.T. treatments lower the risk of cardiovascular disease.

2.Efficient fat loss: By elevating your metabolism and promoting fat oxidation, S.I.T. supports weight loss in a fraction of the time required by traditional methods.

3.Enhanced athletic performance: The explosive nature of S.I.T. improves speed, power, and agility, making it an excellent addition to sports training.

4.Time-saving: With workouts as short as 7 minutes, S.I.T. is perfect for busy individuals.

5.Increased endorphin release: The intensity of S.I.T. stimulates the release of feel-good hormones, reducing stress and enhancing mental clarity.

Who can benefit from S.I.T.?

S.I.T. is an inclusive training method that can benefit a wide range of individuals:

- **Beginners**: Simple, customizable workouts make it easy to start at your own pace.
- **Busy professionals**: Short sessions fit seamlessly into packed schedules.
- **Athletes**: High-intensity sprints build strength, speed, and endurance.
- **Weight-loss seekers**: Its fat-burning capabilities make it a top choice for those aiming to shed pounds.

Limitations and considerations

While S.I.T. offers numerous benefits, it's not without its challenges:

1.Intensity: The all-out effort required can be intimidating, especially for beginners. It's essential to start slowly and build intensity over time.

2.Recovery needs: S.I.T. places a significant strain on the body, making proper recovery crucial to avoid overtraining.

3.Health conditions: Individuals with certain medical conditions, such as heart problems or joint issues, should consult a healthcare provider before attempting S.I.T.

Conclusion

Sprint-Interval Training is a game-changer for modern fitness. It combines intensity, efficiency, and adaptability to deliver unmatched results in minimal time.There is a tried-and-true method to success with S.I.T., whether your goal is to reduce weight, increase strength, or enhance general health.

In the chapters ahead, we'll dive deeper into the mechanics of S.I.T., explore how to structure workouts, and provide practical tips for integrating this powerful method into your daily routine.

Chapter 2: The science behind S.I.T.

Sprint-Interval Training (S.I.T.) is not just a trend; it is rooted in well-established scientific principles and backed by extensive research. Understanding the science behind S.I.T. can deepen our appreciation of why this method is so effective and how it impacts our body. This chapter will explore the physiological mechanisms, metabolic responses, and long-term benefits that make S.I.T. a powerful training strategy.

The basics of energy systems

To understand the science of S.I.T., we must first explore how the body produces energy during exercise. Our muscles rely on three primary energy systems:

1.The ATP-PC system

- This mechanism can power brief, strong bursts of activity that don't last more than ten seconds. It makes use of the energy that the muscles have already stored as phosphocreatine (PC) and adenosine triphosphate (ATP).

- The ATP-PC system is responsible for fuelling the initial burst of intense activity during S.I.T., whether it's a sprint or HIIT.

2.The glycolytic (Anaerobic) system

- This system takes over when the ATP-PC system depletes. It breaks down glucose to produce ATP without requiring oxygen.
- This process generates energy for activities lasting up to 2 minutes but produces lactic acid as a byproduct, leading to muscle fatigue.

3.The oxidative (Aerobic) system

- The oxidative system is slower but sustainable, providing energy for prolonged, lower-intensity exercise by using oxygen to break down carbohydrates, fats, and proteins.
- During the recovery phases of S.I.T., this system works to replenish energy stores and remove waste products like lactic acid.

The role of high-intensity intervals

S.I.T. is unique because it pushes the anaerobic systems (ATP-PC and glycolytic) to their limits. This creates a significant energy demand, triggering several physiological adaptations:

1.Increased mitochondrial density

- ○ Mitochondria generate energy and are so called the "powerhouses" of cells. Research has demonstrated that S.I.T. can enhance the body's energy generation efficiency by increasing mitochondrial density.

2.Enhanced oxygen utilization

- ○ By alternating between intense sprints and recovery, S.I.T. trains the body to use oxygen more effectively, leading to improved aerobic and anaerobic fitness.

3.Greater lactate threshold

- ○ When the rate of lactic acid buildup exceeds the body's ability to eliminate it, a state of exhaustion known as the threshold for lactate is achieved. By raising this barrier, S.I.T. enables users to maintain greater intensities for longer.

Metabolic impact of S.I.T.

S.I.T. significantly influences the body's metabolism, both during and after a workout.

1.Excess post-exercise oxygen consumption (EPOC)

- ○ Peak oxygen consumption (EPOC), sometimes called the "afterburn effect," is a result of prolonged physical exertion.

- ○ The strong EPOC impact that S.I.T. produces means that the body's calorie-burning rate remains increased for hours after the activity. Because of this, it is a very effective strategy for reducing body fat.

2.Fat oxidation

- ○ Research shows that S.I.T. increases fat oxidation during recovery phases and throughout the day, even in shorter sessions. This makes it a powerful tool for reducing body fat.

3.Improved insulin sensitivity

- ○ S.I.T. improves insulin sensitivity, which in turn improves the body's capacity to control blood sugar levels. This effect is particularly beneficial for preventing or managing type 2 diabetes.

Cardiovascular benefits

In terms of heart health, S.I.T. makes a huge difference, challenging the heart and circulatory system in ways traditional steady-state cardio cannot.

1.Increased stroke volume

- The quantity of blood pumped by the heart with each beat is called stroke volume. Stroke volume is improved with regular S.I.T. treatments, which in turn allows the heart to supply oxygen to working muscles more effectively.

2. Lower resting heart rate

- Resting heart rate drops as cardiac efficiency rises, a sign of better cardiovascular fitness.

3. Reduced blood pressure

- Studies have shown that S.I.T. can lower both systolic and diastolic blood pressure, reducing the risk of heart disease.

Hormonal responses

S.I.T. triggers the release of several key hormones that contribute to its effectiveness:

1. Adrenaline and noradrenaline

- These "fight or flight" hormones are released during intense exercise, promoting fat breakdown and increasing energy availability.

2. Growth hormone

- High-intensity exercise stimulates the release of growth hormone, which aids in muscle repair, fat metabolism, and overall recovery.

3. Endorphins

- Often referred to as "feel-good" hormones, endorphins are released during and after S.I.T., reducing stress and improving mood.

S.I.T. and muscle adaptations

While often associated with cardiovascular fitness, S.I.T. also impacts muscular strength and endurance:

1. Fast-twitch muscle fiber recruitment

- S.I.T. primarily targets fast-twitch fibers, responsible for explosive, high-intensity movements. These fibers are essential for power and speed.

2. Improved muscle endurance

- By repeatedly pushing muscles to their limits, S.I.T. enhances endurance and fatigue resistance.

3. Muscle protein synthesis

○ The intense nature of S.I.T. stimulates muscle protein synthesis, promoting repair and growth.

Long-term benefits of S.I.T.

The cumulative effects of S.I.T. extend far beyond short-term results, offering a range of long-term health benefits:

1.Reduced risk of chronic diseases

○ S.I.T. has been linked to lower risks of cardiovascular disease, type 2 diabetes, and metabolic syndrome.

2.Improved brain health

○ High-intensity exercise increases blood flow to the brain, enhancing cognitive function and reducing the risk of neurodegenerative conditions like Alzheimer's disease.

3.Longevity

○ Studies suggest that individuals who engage in high-intensity exercise live longer, healthier lives.

Scientific studies supporting S.I.T.

Numerous studies have demonstrated the efficacy of S.I.T.:

1.Time-efficiency study

○ A landmark study published in *The Journal of Physiology* compared S.I.T. with steady-state cardio. It found that just 10 minutes of S.I.T. (including warm-up and recovery) provided comparable cardiovascular benefits to 50 minutes of steady-state exercise.

2.Fat loss study

○ Research in *Obesity Science & Practice* revealed that participants who performed S.I.T. lost more body fat than those who engaged in traditional cardio, despite spending less total time exercising.

3.Diabetes study

○ A study in *Diabetologia* demonstrated that S.I.T. improved insulin sensitivity by 23% in just two weeks, making it a promising intervention for managing diabetes.

Challenges and considerations

While S.I.T. offers remarkable benefits, it is not without challenges:

1.High intensity

- ○ The all-out effort required can be physically and mentally demanding, especially for beginners. Gradual progression is essential.

2.Recovery needs

- ○ S.I.T. places significant strain on the body, necessitating proper recovery to prevent overtraining and injuries.

3.Individual variability

- ○ Factors such as age, fitness level, and underlying health conditions can influence an individual's ability to perform S.I.T. safely.

Conclusion

The science behind S.I.T. reveals why this training method is so effective. By targeting multiple energy systems, stimulating hormonal responses, and promoting cardiovascular and muscular adaptations, S.I.T. delivers impressive results in a fraction of the time required by traditional workouts.

As we move forward, we'll explore how to harness these scientific principles to design effective S.I.T. workouts that fit your goals and lifestyle.

Chapter 3: The benefits of a 7-minute workout

In today's fast-paced world, the idea of committing to long, grueling workouts can feel daunting. Enter the 7-minute workout—a revolutionary concept that promises maximum results in minimal time. While it might seem too good to be true, science and countless success stories confirm that these brief, high-intensity sessions can deliver significant health and fitness benefits. In this chapter, we'll explore the wide-ranging advantages of a 7-minute workout, from physical and mental health to time efficiency and accessibility.

1.Time efficiency: Fitness for the busy modern lifestyle

One of the most compelling benefits of the 7-minute workout is its time efficiency. For many, lack of time is the primary barrier to regular exercise. A workout that can be completed in just seven minutes eliminates this obstacle, making fitness achievable for even the busiest individuals.

Why seven minutes?

The duration of seven minutes strikes a perfect balance between brevity and intensity. High-intensity interval training (HIIT) principles, which the 7-minute workout follows, show that short bursts of effort can yield the same—or even greater—benefits as longer, moderate-intensity sessions.

Real-life applications

Whether you're a full-time professional, a parent juggling responsibilities, or a student with a packed schedule, finding seven minutes in your day is doable. The workout can be slotted into a lunch break, completed first thing in the morning, or even squeezed in before bed.

2.Accessibility: No gym required

The 7-minute workout doesn't require a gym membership, expensive equipment, or a dedicated workout space. All you need is a small area, a chair, and your body weight.

Benefits of bodyweight training

The exercises in the 7-minute workout are designed to use your body as resistance. Push-ups, squats, and planks effectively target different muscle groups without additional equipment. This makes the workout accessible to people of all fitness levels.

Exercise anywhere, anytime

From hotel rooms to living rooms, the 7-minute workout can be performed virtually anywhere. Its portability ensures that your fitness routine doesn't suffer while traveling or during unexpected schedule changes.

3.Physical health benefits

The 7-minute workout offers a wide range of physical health benefits, proving that you don't need hours at the gym to improve your fitness.

Cardiovascular fitness

High-intensity intervals elevate your heart rate quickly, improving cardiovascular health over time. Regular practice enhances heart strength, blood circulation, and oxygen delivery to muscles.

Fat loss and weight management

Despite its short duration, the 7-minute workout can burn a significant number of calories, especially when performed with maximum effort. Moreover, it triggers excess post-exercise oxygen consumption (EPOC), meaning your body continues to burn calories for hours after the session.

Muscle strength and endurance

The workout incorporates strength-training elements, such as squats, push-ups, and planks, which build muscle strength and endurance. This combination not only sculpts your physique but also supports functional fitness—making everyday tasks easier.

Improved flexibility and mobility

Dynamic movements in the 7-minute workout, like lunges and jumping jacks, enhance flexibility and joint mobility. Over time, this reduces the risk of injuries and improves overall movement quality.

4.Mental health benefits

Exercise has long been recognized for its positive impact on mental health, and the 7-minute workout is no exception.

Stress reduction

The intense bursts of activity in the workout stimulate the release of endorphins, the body's natural "feel-good" hormones. These chemicals help alleviate stress, reduce anxiety, and promote a sense of well-being.

Mood enhancement

Regular exercise has been shown to combat symptoms of depression by boosting serotonin and dopamine levels. The quick nature of the 7-minute workout means you can experience a mental "reset" in a short amount of time.

Improved focus and cognitive function

High-intensity exercise increases blood flow to the brain, improving concentration, memory, and problem-solving abilities. A quick session before tackling a demanding task can enhance productivity and mental clarity.

5.Scalability: Suited for all fitness levels

The 7-minute workout is highly adaptable, making it suitable for beginners and seasoned athletes alike.

For beginners

Newcomers can adjust the intensity by performing modified versions of exercises. For example, push-ups can be done on the knees, and jumping jacks can be replaced with step jacks. The workout's short duration also makes it less intimidating for those new to fitness.

For advanced users

Experienced individuals can increase the intensity by performing faster repetitions, using weights, or adding extra rounds to the session.

Tailored goals

Whether your aim is weight loss, strength building, or improving endurance, the 7-minute workout can be customized to focus on specific objectives.

6.Consistency and habit formation

One of the biggest challenges in fitness is maintaining consistency. The simplicity and brevity of the 7-minute workout make it easier to integrate into daily life.

Breaking the inertia

Starting a workout routine often feels overwhelming, but knowing that it only takes seven minutes removes excuses and lowers the barrier to entry.

Building a routine

Consistency is key to seeing results. With the 7-minute workout, you can establish a daily exercise habit without disrupting your schedule. Over time, this habit can pave the way for more extensive fitness goals.

7.A full-body workout in minutes

The 7-minute workout is strategically designed to target all major muscle groups in a short time.

Upper body

Push-ups and triceps dips strengthen the chest, shoulders, and arms.

Lower body

Squats, lunges, and step-ups engage the glutes, quadriceps, hamstrings, and calves.

Core

Planks and abdominal crunches activate the core muscles, improving stability and posture.

Cardiovascular system

Jumping jacks and high-knee runs elevate the heart rate, delivering a cardio boost.

8.Scientific backing

The 7-minute workout is not just a clever gimmick; it's supported by robust scientific research.

Landmark study

A 2013 study published in the *American College of Sports Medicine's Health & Fitness Journal* demonstrated that high-intensity circuit training, like the 7-minute workout, effectively improves fitness levels and burns fat in a fraction of the time required by traditional methods.

Comparable to longer workouts

Research has shown that short, intense sessions can produce the same cardiovascular and metabolic benefits as longer workouts, such as jogging for 30–60 minutes.

Improved insulin sensitivity

Studies also highlight that even brief HIIT-style workouts enhance the body's insulin sensitivity, reducing the risk of type 2 diabetes.

9.Cost-effective and sustainable

The 7-minute workout eliminates many financial and logistical barriers to fitness.

No gym memberships

You don't need a gym membership, expensive equipment, or personal trainers to benefit.

Sustainability

The workout's minimal requirements make it easy to sustain over the long term, ensuring consistency and adherence.

10.Results in less time

Perhaps the most attractive benefit of the 7-minute workout is its ability to deliver results in a short time.

Fat loss

Consistent practice, paired with proper nutrition, can lead to noticeable weight loss and body composition improvements.

Increased strength and stamina

The workout's combination of strength and cardio exercises builds muscular endurance and boosts stamina.

Improved overall health

With regular practice, you'll notice better energy levels, reduced stress, and an overall sense of vitality.

Conclusion

The 7-minute workout is a perfect solution for those who want to prioritize their health without sacrificing time. By combining time efficiency, accessibility, and a wide range of physical and mental health benefits, it makes fitness achievable for everyone.

In the next chapter, we'll dive into how to structure an effective 7-minute workout and provide practical tips to maximize its potential.

Chapter 4: Building an effective workout

Creating an effective workout is about more than just stringing together random exercises. It requires a thoughtful approach to ensure the workout aligns with your goals, is safe, and is engaging enough to maintain consistency. In this chapter, we will explore the key principles of designing an effective workout, discuss the importance of variety, and offer practical steps to help you create a routine that works for you—whether it's a 7-minute session or a longer training block.

1.Define your goals

Every effective workout begins with a clear understanding of your fitness goals. These goals will determine the structure, intensity, and type of exercises in your routine.

Common goals

1.Weight loss

- Focus on high-intensity interval training (HIIT) and exercises that engage multiple muscle groups to maximize calorie burn.

2.Muscle building

- Prioritize resistance training with progressive overload, using bodyweight or external weights.

3.Improved endurance

- Incorporate aerobic exercises and activities that challenge cardiovascular fitness.

4.Increased flexibility and mobility

- Add dynamic stretches, yoga, or Pilates-inspired movements to enhance range of motion.

5.General health

- Balance cardio, strength, and flexibility exercises to promote overall well-being.

2.The principles of workout design

To build an effective workout, it's essential to understand the foundational principles of exercise design.

A.Specificity

The exercises you choose should directly support your fitness goals. For example, if you want to improve your sprinting speed, prioritize lower-body power exercises like squats and lunges.

B.Progressive overload

To see improvements, you must gradually challenge your body. This can be achieved by increasing resistance, performing more repetitions, or reducing rest time between sets.

C.Balance

An effective workout addresses all major muscle groups to ensure balanced strength and reduce the risk of injury. Avoid overtraining specific areas while neglecting others.

D.Rest and recovery

Adequate rest between exercises and workout sessions is crucial for muscle repair, growth, and performance. Rest periods depend on the intensity of the workout and your fitness level.

E.Variation

Changing up your routine prevents plateaus and keeps your workouts engaging. Variety in exercises, intensity, and duration ensures consistent progress.

3.Structuring a workout

An effective workout is more than just a list of exercises; it follows a logical progression to maximize results and minimize risk.

A.Warm-up (5–10 Minutes)

A proper warm-up prepares your body for exercise by increasing heart rate, improving circulation, and loosening muscles. Examples include:

- Light cardio: Jogging in place or jumping jacks.
- Dynamic stretches: Leg swings, arm circles, or hip openers.

B.Main workout (15–45 Minutes)

The core of your session depends on your goals and fitness level.

1.Circuit training

- Ideal for 7-minute workouts, this method involves performing a series of exercises targeting different muscle groups with minimal rest between sets.
- Example: Push-ups → Squats → Plank → Jumping Jacks.

2.Strength training

- Focus on resistance exercises to build muscle.
- Example: Bodyweight lunges, push-ups, and planks with added difficulty over time.

3.Cardio intervals

- Alternate between high- and low-intensity exercises to boost cardiovascular fitness.
- Example: Sprinting for 30 seconds, walking for 1 minute (repeat for 15 minutes).

C.Cool down (5–10 Minutes)

The cool-down is essential for bringing your heart rate back to normal and reducing muscle soreness. It may include:

- Light stretching: Focus on major muscle groups.
- Breathing exercises: Help regulate your nervous system post-workout.

4.Choosing the right exercises

The exercises in your routine should be selected based on your goals, fitness level, and preferences.

A.Compound vs. isolation exercises

- **Compound exercises:** Target multiple muscle groups at once, making them ideal for time-efficient workouts. Examples: Squats, push-ups, and burpees.
- **Isolation exercises:** Focus on a single muscle group. Useful for targeting weaknesses or specific areas. Examples: Bicep curls, tricep dips.

B.Functional movements

Incorporating functional exercises improves your ability to perform everyday tasks. Examples: Deadlifts mimic lifting objects off the ground, while lunges replicate walking upstairs.

C.Bodyweight vs. equipment-based workouts

- Bodyweight exercises are accessible and versatile, requiring no equipment.
- Adding equipment like resistance bands, dumbbells, or kettlebells can increase difficulty and provide variety.

5.Adapting for fitness levels

An effective workout should be challenging but manageable. Tailoring the intensity ensures you stay motivated and avoid injury.

A.Beginner modifications

- Reduce the number of repetitions.
- Perform exercises at a slower pace.
- Use support, such as a wall or chair, for balance.

B.Advanced variations

- Add weight or resistance.
- Perform explosive movements (e.g., jump squats).
- Decrease rest time between exercises.

6.Keeping workouts engaging

Consistency is key to achieving results, and boredom is one of the biggest obstacles to staying on track.

A.Variety

Change your routine every 4–6 weeks to keep things fresh. Experiment with different exercise styles, such as yoga, Pilates, or dance-inspired workouts.

B.Tracking progress

Keeping a workout journal or using a fitness app allows you to monitor improvements and set new goals.

C.Partner or group workouts

Exercising with a friend or joining a class can boost motivation and accountability.

7.Safety considerations

Safety is paramount when building and performing a workout.

A.Proper form

Always prioritize correct technique over speed or weight. Poor form increases the risk of injury and reduces effectiveness.

B.Listen to your body

Avoid pushing through pain or fatigue. Modify or skip exercises if necessary.

C.Medical clearance

If you're new to exercise or have preexisting health conditions, consult a healthcare professional before starting a new routine.

8.Sample 7-minute workout

Here's a sample 7-minute workout designed to target all major muscle groups:

1. Jumping Jacks (30 seconds) – Warm-up and cardio.

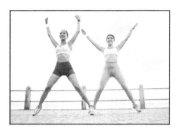

2. Wall Sit (30 seconds) – Lower-body strength.

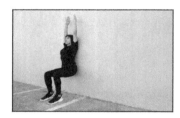

3. Push-Ups (30 seconds) – Upper-body strength.

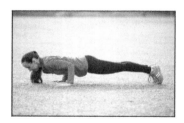

4. Abdominal Crunches (30 seconds) – Core strength.

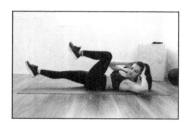

5. Step-Ups on Chair (30 seconds) – Lower body and cardio.

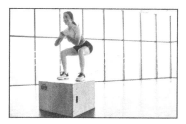

6. Squats (30 seconds) – Full-body strength.

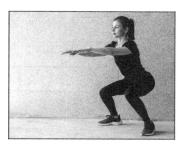

7. Plank (30 seconds) – Core stability.

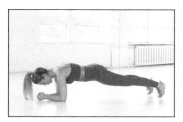

Repeat as needed for a longer session.

9.The role of recovery

Recovery is an often-overlooked but critical part of any effective workout plan.

A.Active recovery

Engage in light activities like walking or yoga on rest days to promote circulation and muscle repair.

B.Nutrition and hydration

Fuel your body with balanced meals and stay hydrated to optimize performance and recovery.

C.Sleep

Adequate sleep is essential for muscle repair, hormone regulation, and overall recovery.

10.Adjusting over time

As your fitness improves, your workout should evolve to keep challenging your body. Gradual progression ensures continued results and keeps you motivated.

A.Increase intensity

Add weight, increase reps, or shorter rest periods.

B.Incorporate new exercises

Introduce movements that challenge your body in different ways.

C.Reassess goals

As you achieve milestones, set new objectives to stay focused and driven.

Conclusion

Building an effective workout requires planning, intention, and adaptability. By understanding your goals, incorporating variety, and adhering to key exercise principles, you can create a routine that not only delivers results but also fits seamlessly into your life. In the next chapter, we'll discuss the importance of consistency and how to maintain motivation on your fitness journey.

Chapter 5: Why home workouts?

Home workouts have become a cornerstone of modern fitness, offering convenience, accessibility, and flexibility for people of all fitness levels. Whether you're a busy professional, a parent juggling family responsibilities, or someone looking to save time and money, working out at home is an effective and sustainable solution. In this chapter, we'll explore the many reasons why home workouts are gaining popularity and delve into their advantages over traditional gym-based routines.

1.Convenience: Fitness on your terms

One of the most appealing aspects of home workouts is their unmatched convenience.

No commute required

Traditional gyms often require travel time that can eat into your day. With home workouts, your exercise space is just a few steps away, making it easier to integrate fitness into your daily routine.

Flexibility in timing

Unlike gym schedules or fitness classes, home workouts allow you to exercise whenever it suits you. Whether it's an early morning session, a mid-day break, or a late-night sweat, your workout fits seamlessly into your lifestyle.

Weather-proof fitness

Rain, snow, or heat waves won't disrupt your home workout plans. You can maintain consistency regardless of external conditions.

2.Cost-effectiveness

Gym memberships, fitness classes, and personal trainers can be expensive. Home workouts provide an affordable alternative.

No membership fees

Working out at home eliminates recurring costs. Once you invest in basic equipment (if needed), your workouts are essentially free.

Minimal equipment required

Many home workouts, including bodyweight exercises, require little to no equipment. Items like resistance bands, dumbbells, or yoga mats are affordable and versatile additions to your setup.

Saving on extras

Home workouts also save money on travel expenses, childcare costs, and gym attire. There's no need for fancy workout clothes when you're exercising in your living room!

3.Time efficiency

Time is a valuable commodity, and home workouts maximize efficiency by eliminating common time-consuming barriers.

No waiting for equipment

In a crowded gym, waiting for machines or weights can disrupt your flow. At home, you're in control of the pace and progression of your workout.

Short workouts, big results

Home workouts often emphasize high-intensity, short-duration routines like the 7-minute workout. These efficient formats ensure you can achieve significant results in less time.

Customizable sessions

Whether you have 10 minutes or an hour, home workouts can be tailored to fit your schedule, ensuring you stay active even on the busiest days.

4.Privacy and comfort

For many, the gym can feel intimidating or overwhelming. Home workouts provide a private and comfortable environment.

Judgment-free zone

At home, there's no pressure to look a certain way or compare yourself to others. You can focus solely on your fitness journey without distractions or self-consciousness.

Personalized space

Your home workout space can be as simple or elaborate as you like. Whether it's a corner of your living room or a dedicated home gym, you can create an environment that suits your preferences.

Freedom to experiment

Home workouts allow you to try new exercises, experiment with routines, or practice yoga poses without fear of making mistakes in front of others.

5.Accessibility for all

Home workouts remove many of the barriers that prevent people from exercising regularly.

For beginners

Starting a fitness journey at home can feel less intimidating than joining a gym. Beginners can learn and grow at their own pace with online resources and beginner-friendly routines.

For busy parents

Parents often struggle to find time for the gym due to childcare responsibilities. Home workouts allow parents to stay active while keeping an eye on their children.

For people with disabilities or injuries

Home workouts can be customized to accommodate physical limitations, ensuring everyone has access to effective exercise options.

6.Variety and customization

Home workouts are incredibly versatile, offering endless possibilities to keep your routine fresh and engaging.

Exercise styles

From strength training and cardio to yoga and Pilates, home workouts encompass a wide range of exercise styles.

Online resources

The internet is a treasure trove of workout videos, apps, and guides, catering to every fitness goal and preference. Platforms like YouTube, fitness apps, and streaming services provide professional guidance at no cost or for a small fee.

Tailored routines

At home, you have the freedom to customize your workouts based on your goals, preferences, and available time. This flexibility ensures you stay motivated and consistent.

7.Maintaining consistency

Consistency is key to achieving fitness goals, and home workouts make it easier to maintain regular exercise habits.

Fewer excuses

Proximity and convenience mean you're less likely to skip a workout. Without the need to commute or adhere to gym hours, exercising becomes a more straightforward part of your daily routine.

Building a habit

A regular workout space at home can serve as a visual reminder to stay active. Over time, exercising at home becomes an ingrained habit.

Adaptable to life changes

Whether you're dealing with a busy schedule, unexpected travel, or seasonal changes, home workouts adapt to your life, helping you stay consistent.

8.Reducing stress and enhancing mental health

Exercising at home offers mental health benefits beyond the physical advantages.

Creating a sanctuary

Your home workout space can become a sanctuary for self-care. With calming music or soothing lighting, it's a place to unwind and focus on your well-being.

Stress relief

Exercise is a proven stress reliever, and the convenience of home workouts ensures you can de-stress whenever needed, without the additional hassle of going to a gym.

Improved focus and productivity

Taking a short workout break at home can rejuvenate your mind, improve focus, and enhance productivity, especially for those working remotely.

9.The rise of virtual fitness communities

Despite the solitary nature of home workouts, virtual communities have made it possible to stay connected and motivated.

Online classes and challenges

Live-streamed classes and fitness challenges foster a sense of community and accountability. Participants can connect with others, share progress, and stay motivated.

Social media inspiration

Platforms like Instagram and TikTok provide inspiration, tips, and a platform to celebrate milestones with like-minded individuals.

Personalized coaching

Many fitness apps and online programs offer personalized coaching and feedback, blending the benefits of home workouts with professional guidance.

10.Environmental and ethical benefits

Choosing to work out at home can align with sustainable and ethical values.

Reduced carbon footprint

By eliminating commutes to the gym, home workouts contribute to lower carbon emissions, making them an environmentally friendly choice.

Support for small businesses

Many independent trainers and creators offer online classes or programs, allowing you to support small businesses and individuals.

11.Overcoming challenges of home workouts

While the benefits of home workouts are numerous, there are challenges to consider. Recognizing these obstacles and finding solutions ensures long-term success.

Limited space

- Solution: Choose bodyweight exercises or use portable equipment like resistance bands.
- Adapt by clearing a small area or rearranging furniture temporarily.

Motivation

- Solution: Set specific goals, follow structured programs, or involve friends and family for accountability.

Distractions

- Solution: Schedule dedicated workout times and create a designated space for exercise to minimize interruptions.

Conclusion

Home workouts offer unparalleled convenience, accessibility, and flexibility, making them an excellent option for people from all walks of life. By removing barriers such as time, cost, and intimidation, they empower individuals to take control of their fitness journeys. Whether you're a beginner seeking to start small or an experienced athlete looking to supplement your routine, home workouts provide endless opportunities to achieve your health and wellness goals.

In the next chapter, we'll discuss how to set up your perfect home workout space, ensuring you have everything you need to succeed.

Chapter 6: S.I.T. vs. HIIT

In the world of fitness, acronyms like S.I.T. (Sprint Interval Training) and HIIT (High-Intensity Interval Training) dominate the conversation. Both approaches are celebrated for their ability to deliver impressive results in less time than traditional workouts. However, while S.I.T. and HIIT share similarities, they cater to different needs, goals, and fitness levels. This chapter dives into the distinctions and overlaps between these two training methods, helping you decide which is best suited for your fitness journey.

1.Understanding S.I.T. (Sprint Interval Training)

Sprint Interval Training is a specific subset of interval training that emphasizes short bursts of maximum effort, typically through sprints or similarly explosive movements, followed by extended recovery periods.

Key characteristics of S.I.T.

- **Intensity:** Near-maximal to maximal effort, typically at 90-100% of your capacity.
- **Duration:** Very short work intervals (e.g., 10-30 seconds).
- **Recovery:** Longer recovery periods, often at a low intensity or complete rest (e.g., 1-4 minutes).
- **Focus:** Prioritizes anaerobic energy systems, building power and speed.

Example S.I.T. session

- Sprint at full speed for 20 seconds.
- Walk or rest for 2 minutes.
- Repeat for 6-8 cycles.

S.I.T. workouts are designed to push your body to its limit in brief intervals, making it a time-efficient way to improve athletic performance and cardiovascular fitness.

2.Understanding HIIT (High-Intensity Interval Training)

High-Intensity Interval Training is a broader training methodology that alternates between periods of high-intensity effort and short recovery or lower-intensity activity.

Key characteristics of HIIT

- **Intensity:** High effort, usually at 70-90% of your capacity.
- **Duration:** Work intervals typically last 20 seconds to 1 minute.
- **Recovery:** Shorter recovery periods compared to S.I.T., often active recovery (e.g., jogging or light movement).
- **Focus:** Combines aerobic and anaerobic systems, improving endurance, strength, and overall fitness.

Example HIIT session

- Jump squats for 30 seconds.
- Jog or walk for 15 seconds.
- Repeat with different exercises for 15-20 minutes.

HIIT is a versatile workout style that can incorporate various exercises, such as bodyweight movements, cycling, or resistance training, making it accessible to a wide audience.

3.Comparing S.I.T. and HIIT

While S.I.T. and HIIT share a foundation in interval training, their differences lie in intensity, recovery, and overall application.

A.Intensity levels

- **S.I.T.:** Requires maximum effort, which can feel more taxing on the body.
- **HIIT:** Demands high effort but allows for a broader range of intensities, making it more manageable for beginners.

B.Duration of work and recovery

- **S.I.T.:** Short work intervals with long recovery periods to ensure maximum performance during sprints.
- **HIIT:** Longer work intervals with shorter recovery, keeping the heart rate elevated throughout the session.

C.Energy systems utilized

- **S.I.T.:** Primarily anaerobic, focusing on short bursts of power and speed.
- **HIIT:** A mix of anaerobic and aerobic systems, targeting endurance and calorie burn.

D.Overall time commitment

- **S.I.T.:** Shorter sessions due to the intense nature, typically 10-20 minutes.
- **HIIT:** Longer sessions, ranging from 15-30 minutes, due to slightly lower intensity.

E.Suitability for goals

- **S.I.T.:** Ideal for athletes or those seeking explosive power and improved sprinting ability.
- **HIIT:** Better suited for general fitness, weight loss, and cardiovascular health.

4.Benefits of S.I.T.

S.I.T. is not just for elite athletes; it offers significant benefits for anyone looking to optimize their fitness.

A.Time efficiency

S.I.T. packs a powerful punch in a short amount of time, making it ideal for busy schedules.

B.Improved anaerobic capacity

By pushing your body to its limits, S.I.T. enhances your ability to perform high-intensity activities without fatiguing as quickly.

C.Enhanced athletic performance

S.I.T. builds speed, power, and agility, making it a favorite among athletes.

D.Fat loss

Like HIIT, S.I.T. triggers excess post-exercise oxygen consumption (EPOC), leading to continued calorie burn after the workout.

E.Cardiovascular health

Research shows that S.I.T. can improve heart health and endurance, even with minimal time commitment.

---

5. Benefits of HIIT

HIIT's versatility and accessibility make it a popular choice for people with diverse fitness goals.

A.Calorie burn and fat loss

HIIT burns calories during the workout and afterward, thanks to the EPOC effect.

B.Improved endurance

The mix of high-intensity and lower-intensity periods enhances both aerobic and anaerobic capacity.

C.Versatility

HIIT can incorporate a variety of exercises, including bodyweight, strength, and cardio movements, keeping workouts engaging.

D.Accessibility

HIIT is suitable for all fitness levels, as the intensity can be adjusted to match individual capabilities.

E.Health benefits

HIIT has been shown to improve blood pressure, insulin sensitivity, and overall cardiovascular health.

6.Choosing between S.I.T. and HIIT

Your choice between S.I.T. and HIIT depends on several factors, including your goals, fitness level, and personal preferences.

A.Goals

- Choose **S.I.T.** if your focus is on building power, speed, or athletic performance.
- Opt for **HIIT** if you're aiming for general fitness, weight loss, or endurance.

B.Fitness level

- **Beginners:** HIIT is more forgiving, as it allows for moderate effort and shorter recovery periods.
- **Advanced athletes:** S.I.T. is more challenging and ideal for those seeking maximum performance.

C.Time availability

- If you're pressed for time, S.I.T.'s shorter sessions might be more appealing.
- For a more balanced workout, HIIT provides variety and a slightly longer duration.

D.Enjoyment

The best workout is the one you'll stick with. Try both methods and see which resonates more with your preferences and lifestyle.

7.Combining S.I.T. and HIIT

For those who want the best of both worlds, combining S.I.T. and HIIT can create a well-rounded fitness routine.

Example hybrid workout

1.S.I.T. Segment:

- ○ Sprint at maximum effort for 15 seconds.
- ○ Rest for 1 minute.
- ○ Repeat for 4 cycles.

2.HIIT Segment:

- ○ 30 seconds of jump squats.
- ○ 15 seconds of rest.
- ○ 30 seconds of push-ups.
- ○ 15 seconds of rest.
- ○ Repeat for 3 cycles.

This approach leverages the explosive power of S.I.T. with the endurance and variety of HIIT.

8.Common misconceptions

A.S.I.T. is only for athletes

While it's true that S.I.T. is demanding, beginners can adapt by starting with lower intensity and building up over time.

B.HIIT and S.I.T. are the same

Although they share similarities, their differences in intensity, recovery, and application set them apart.

C.Longer workouts are better

Both S.I.T. and HIIT prove that short, focused sessions can be more effective than lengthy, moderate-intensity workouts.

9.Scientific evidence

Both S.I.T. and HIIT have been extensively studied for their effectiveness.

- **S.I.T.**   **studies:**
  Research shows that just a few minutes of S.I.T. per week can improve VO2 max and anaerobic capacity, rivaling longer endurance workouts.
- **HIIT**   **studies:**
  HIIT has been linked to improved metabolic health, fat loss, and cardiovascular fitness, making it a favorite among researchers and trainers.

Conclusion

Both S.I.T. and HIIT offer powerful, time-efficient ways to improve fitness, burn calories, and boost overall health. While S.I.T. emphasizes explosive power and maximal effort, HIIT provides versatility and accessibility for a wide audience. The choice ultimately depends on your goals, fitness level, and personal preferences. With the flexibility to combine or alternate between the two, you can create a dynamic and engaging workout routine that keeps you motivated and delivers results.

In the next chapter, we'll explore how to set goals and track progress to maximize the benefits of your S.I.T. and HIIT workouts.

Chapter 7: Getting ready for success

Success in fitness—and in life—often hinges on preparation. Whether you're starting a new workout routine or striving for a healthier lifestyle, setting the stage for success is crucial. This chapter explores the practical steps, mindset shifts, and strategies you need to get ready for a sustainable and rewarding fitness journey. From planning your workout space to building the right mindset, these tips will help you start strong and stay consistent.

1.Define your goals

Before you dive into a fitness routine, it's essential to define what success means to you. Having clear, specific goals provides motivation and a sense of direction.

A.Be specific

- Vague goals like "get fit" or "lose weight" are harder to measure. Instead, set specific objectives like:
    - "Lose 10 pounds in 3 months."
    - "Run a 5K by the end of the year."
    - "Complete a 7-minute S.I.T. workout daily for 30 days."

B.Use the SMART framework

Goals should be:

- **Specific:** Clear and well-defined.
- **Measurable:** Quantifiable to track progress.
- **Achievable:** Realistic given your starting point.
- **Relevant:** Aligned with your priorities.
- **Time-bound:** Set within a deadline to maintain focus.

C.Short-term vs. long-term goals

Set a mix of short-term goals (e.g., improving flexibility in a month) and long-term aspirations (e.g., building lifelong fitness habits).

2.Create a plan

A well-thought-out plan increases the likelihood of sticking to your fitness routine.

A.Choose the right program

Select a workout program that aligns with your goals, fitness level, and schedule. For example:

- If time is limited, opt for a 7-minute S.I.T. routine.
- If weight loss is your priority, include high-intensity or calorie-burning exercises.

B.Schedule your workouts

Consistency is key. Treat your workouts as appointments by blocking time in your calendar.

- Morning workouts can set a positive tone for the day.
- Evening sessions might be better for unwinding after work.

C.Plan your rest days

Recovery is as important as exercise. Incorporate rest days to prevent burnout and reduce the risk of injury.

3.Set up your space

Your environment plays a significant role in shaping habits. A well-prepared workout space can inspire consistency and focus.

A.Find the right spot

Choose a space in your home that's:

- Spacious enough for your movements.
- Free of distractions.
- Well-ventilated and comfortable.

B.Gather your equipment

Depending on your routine, you may need:

- A yoga mat or exercise mat.
- Dumbbells, resistance bands, or kettlebells.
- A timer for interval training.
- A sturdy chair for modifications or stability exercises.

C.Organize your space

Keep your workout area tidy and accessible. Seeing your equipment regularly can serve as a reminder to stay active.

4.Build the right mindset

Physical preparation is only half the battle. A strong, resilient mindset is vital for overcoming challenges and staying consistent.

A.Embrace progress over perfection

- Fitness is a journey, not a race. Celebrate small wins, like completing a workout or improving your form.
- Accept setbacks as part of the process and use them as learning opportunities.

B.Focus on intrinsic motivation

While external rewards (like weight loss or compliments) are motivating, internal motivators (like feeling energized or reducing stress) provide lasting commitment.

C.Develop a growth mindset

- Believe in your ability to improve with effort and consistency.
- View challenges as opportunities to grow rather than obstacles.

5.Prepare for obstacles

Every fitness journey faces roadblocks, but anticipating and planning for them can help you stay on track.

A.Time constraints

- Plan shorter, high-intensity workouts like S.I.T. sessions.
- Incorporate "movement snacks" throughout the day, such as quick stretches or a walk.

B.Lack of motivation

- Create a playlist of energizing music.
- Keep inspirational quotes or reminders in your workout space.
- Remember your "why" – the reason you started your fitness journey.

C.Injury or fatigue

- Listen to your body and prioritize rest when needed.
- Modify exercises to accommodate your physical condition.

D.distractions

- Set boundaries during workout time. Communicate with family or roommates about your schedule.
- Turn off notifications on your devices to focus fully on your session.

6.Nutrition and hydration

Fueling your body properly enhances performance and recovery.

A.Balanced diet

- Prioritize whole, nutrient-dense foods like fruits, vegetables, lean proteins, and whole grains.
- Avoid processed foods and sugary snacks, which can cause energy crashes.

B.Timing your meals

- Eat a light snack with carbohydrates and protein 1-2 hours before exercising.
- Refuel post-workout with a mix of protein and carbohydrates to aid recovery.

C.Stay hydrated

- Drink water throughout the day and during your workouts.
- Consider electrolyte-rich beverages if your sessions are intense or last longer than an hour.

7.Tracking progress

Monitoring your progress keeps you motivated and helps you make necessary adjustments.

A.Keep a fitness journal

- Record your workouts, including exercises, duration, and intensity.
- Note how you feel after each session to identify patterns or improvements.

B.Use technology

- Fitness apps or wearable devices can track metrics like heart rate, calories burned, and steps taken.
- Use interval timers or S.I.T.-specific apps to structure your workouts effectively.

C.Take measurements

- Use body measurements, photos, or strength tests to track changes over time.
- Focus on non-scale victories, such as improved energy levels or better posture.

8.Build a support system

A strong support network can make your fitness journey more enjoyable and sustainable.

A.Involve friends and family

- Share your goals with loved ones to create accountability.
- Invite friends to join your workouts for added motivation.

B.Join online communities

- Engage with fitness groups on social media or apps to exchange tips, encouragement, and inspiration.

C.Consider professional guidance

- If you're unsure where to start, hire a personal trainer or follow guided programs online.

9.Celebrate your successes

Acknowledging your progress keeps you motivated and reinforces positive habits.

A.Reward yourself

- Treat yourself to new workout gear, a healthy meal, or a relaxing activity after achieving milestones.

B.Reflect on your achievements

- Take time to appreciate how far you've come, whether it's lifting heavier weights or sticking to your routine for a month.

10.Commit to lifelong learning

Fitness is an evolving journey. Stay open to new techniques, exercises, and approaches to keep your routine fresh and effective.

A. Experiment with Variations

- Mix up your S.I.T. workouts with new exercises to challenge your body.

B.Stay informed

- Read books, follow experts, and attend workshops to deepen your understanding of fitness and health.

Conclusion

Getting ready for success involves more than just choosing a workout—it's about creating an environment, mindset, and routine that support your goals. By defining clear objectives, planning effectively, and building a resilient mindset, you're setting yourself up for long-term fitness success. With preparation as your foundation, you can confidently embark on your fitness journey and tackle challenges with determination.

In the next chapter, we'll explore how to set up the perfect 7-minute S.I.T. workout and make it a cornerstone of your fitness routine.

Chapter 8: The time factor: Why 7 minutes?

In today's fast-paced world, finding time for fitness can feel like an uphill battle. Between work, family commitments, and personal responsibilities, many people struggle to dedicate an hour—or even half an hour—to a traditional workout. Enter the 7-minute workout, a game-changing approach to fitness that prioritizes efficiency without sacrificing effectiveness. But why 7 minutes? What makes this timeframe so appealing, and how does it deliver tangible results?

This chapter explores the science, psychology, and practicality behind the 7-minute workout, illustrating why it's more than just a trend—it's a powerful solution for modern lifestyles.

1.The origins of the 7-minute workout

The 7-minute workout gained global attention in 2013 when researchers Brett Klika and Chris Jordan published their findings in the *American College of Sports Medicine's Health & Fitness Journal*. They introduced a high-intensity circuit training (HICT) protocol designed to deliver maximum benefits in minimal time.

Key features of the original 7-minute workout

- A series of 12 bodyweight exercises targeting major muscle groups.
- Each exercise performed for 30 seconds, with 10 seconds of rest between.
- Exercises arranged to alternate between upper-body, lower-body, and core movements to maximize efficiency.

The concept was simple: by maintaining high intensity and focusing on large muscle groups, you could achieve the same benefits as a longer workout in just 7 minutes.

2.The science behind short workouts

The success of the 7-minute workout isn't just about convenience—it's rooted in scientific principles that demonstrate how short, intense exercise sessions can transform your fitness.

A.The role of high-intensity interval training (HIIT)

The 7-minute workout is a form of HIIT, which alternates between bursts of intense activity and brief rest periods. HIIT has been extensively studied and is proven to:

- Increase cardiovascular fitness.
- Improve metabolic health.
- Enhance fat burning during and after exercise.

B.The power of EPOC (Excess Post-Exercise Oxygen Consumption)

Intense exercise triggers EPOC, commonly known as the "afterburn effect." After a high-intensity workout, your body continues to burn calories as it recovers, increasing the total energy expenditure. A well-structured 7-minute workout can leverage EPOC to extend calorie burn long after the session ends.

C.Muscle engagement and efficiency

The 7-minute format is designed to target multiple muscle groups in quick succession. This approach maximizes workout efficiency by combining strength and cardio benefits in a compact timeframe.

3.Why 7 minutes? The psychological appeal

The specific length of 7 minutes isn't arbitrary—it's a sweet spot that balances effectiveness with accessibility.

A.Breaking down barriers

Many people cite lack of time as the primary reason for skipping exercise. The 7-minute workout eliminates this excuse, making fitness feel achievable even on the busiest days.

B.Low commitment, high return

Committing to 7 minutes feels manageable and non-intimidating. Psychologically, it's easier to motivate yourself for a brief session than a longer workout, reducing the likelihood of procrastination.

C.Habit formation

Short workouts are easier to integrate into daily routines, increasing consistency. Over time, these small, consistent efforts compound, leading to significant fitness improvements.

4.The practical benefits of a 7-minute workout

The practicality of the 7-minute workout is one of its strongest selling points.

A.Time efficiency

- In just 7 minutes, you can complete a full-body workout, targeting strength, endurance, and cardiovascular health.
- Ideal for people with packed schedules, allowing them to stay active without compromising other commitments.

B.Minimal equipment

- Most 7-minute workouts rely on bodyweight exercises, making them accessible to anyone, anywhere.
- All you need is a timer, a chair, and a small space.

C.Versatility

- The format can be adapted to various fitness levels, from beginners to advanced athletes.
- Exercises can be modified or intensified to suit individual needs.

D.Cost-effectiveness

- No gym membership or expensive equipment is required, making the workout financially accessible.

5.Can 7 minutes really be enough?

A common question is whether a 7-minute workout is truly sufficient for fitness gains. The answer depends on your goals, intensity, and consistency.

A.For general fitness

Research supports the effectiveness of short, high-intensity workouts for improving cardiovascular health, muscle strength, and metabolic function.

B.For weight loss

While 7 minutes alone may not create a significant calorie deficit, it can jumpstart fat burning and complement other lifestyle changes, such as improved nutrition.

C.For athletic performance

Athletes may require longer or more specialized training. However, a 7-minute workout can be a valuable addition to cross-training or active recovery days.

D.As a gateway to more activity

For many, the 7-minute workout serves as an entry point to a more active lifestyle. Once the habit is established, individuals often progress to longer or more varied routines.

6.Optimizing your 7-minute workout

To maximize the benefits of a 7-minute workout, it's important to approach it with intention and effort.

A.Focus on intensity

The workout is only effective if you push yourself during the work intervals. Aim for 80-90% of your maximum effort.

B.Prioritize form

Maintaining proper form prevents injuries and ensures you're targeting the right muscles. Take a moment to learn the exercises before diving in.

C.Warm up and cool down

While the workout itself is brief, dedicating a few minutes to warming up and cooling down can enhance performance and recovery.

D.Track your progress

Keep a record of your workouts to monitor improvements in strength, endurance, and consistency.

7.The 7-minute workout as a lifestyle tool

The beauty of the 7-minute workout lies in its adaptability. It's not just a standalone routine—it's a tool you can use to enhance your lifestyle.

A.On busy days

When life gets hectic, a quick 7-minute session ensures you still prioritize your health.

B.As a supplement

Use the 7-minute workout to complement other forms of exercise, such as yoga, running, or weightlifting.

C.Travel-friendly fitness

The minimal equipment and short duration make it perfect for maintaining fitness while traveling.

D.Family-friendly exercise

The simplicity of the workout makes it easy to involve family members, fostering a culture of health and wellness at home.

8.Real-life success stories

Many people have transformed their health and fitness with the 7-minute workout. Here are some examples of its impact:

- **Sarah, a busy mom:** Balancing work and parenting left little time for exercise. The 7-minute workout helped her regain energy and strength without disrupting her schedule.
- **Mark, a frequent traveler:** Mark used the workout to stay consistent during business trips, maintaining his fitness goals despite a demanding travel schedule.
- **Emma, a fitness beginner:** As someone new to exercise, Emma found the 7-minute workout approachable and gradually built confidence and endurance.

9.Common misconceptions

While the 7-minute workout is effective, it's important to address some common misconceptions:

- "It's too short to matter."
  Research proves that intensity matters more than duration in short workouts.
- "It's only for beginners."
  Advanced fitness enthusiasts can increase the intensity or add weights for a greater challenge.
- "It replaces all other workouts."
  While beneficial, the 7-minute workout works best when combined with other activities or used as part of a balanced fitness plan.

Conclusion

The 7-minute workout is more than just a fitness fad—it's a revolutionary approach to exercise that aligns with the demands of modern life. By combining high intensity, strategic design, and psychological appeal, it offers a practical solution for staying active in the face of time constraints. Whether you're a beginner looking to start small or an experienced athlete seeking efficiency, the 7-minute workout proves that even brief efforts can yield significant results.

In the next chapter, we'll explore the different types of S.I.T. workouts and how to tailor them to your goals and preferences.

Chapter 9: Exercises for the 7-minute S.I.T. workout

In this chapter, we will explore the specific exercises that make up a 7-minute S.I.T. (Short Interval Training) workout. This section will guide you through each movement, providing explanations on form, benefits, and how they contribute to an overall effective workout. A proper balance of exercises targeting strength, endurance, and cardiovascular fitness is key to the success of any high-intensity interval training (HIIT) routine. The exercises outlined here are designed to work your entire body in just seven minutes.

1.Jumping jacks

Target area: Full body, with an emphasis on the cardiovascular system.

Jumping jacks are one of the most basic but effective cardio exercises. They work your legs, arms, and core while raising your heart rate, making them an excellent warm-up or full-body movement.

Execution:

- Start with your feet together and arms by your sides.
- Jump your feet out wide while raising your arms overhead.
- Jump back to the starting position.
- Keep a steady rhythm, and try to avoid letting your lower back arch.

Benefits: Jumping jacks help increase your heart rate, improve coordination, and activate multiple muscle groups. As a cardio move, they are perfect for improving endurance and promoting fat loss.

2.Squats

Target area: Legs (quads, hamstrings, and glutes) and core.

Squats are one of the best bodyweight exercises for building strength in your lower body. They primarily target the legs but also engage your core for stability.

Execution:

- Stand with your feet shoulder-width apart.
- Lower your body by bending your knees and pushing your hips back, as though sitting in a chair.
- Keep your chest up and your knees aligned with your toes.
- Return to the standing position by pushing through your heels.

Benefits: Squats are an excellent exercise for building leg strength and endurance. They engage large muscle groups and help improve your mobility and balance. Additionally, they contribute to a higher metabolic rate due to the large muscles involved.

3.Push-ups

Target area: Chest, shoulders, triceps, and core.

Push-ups are a classic upper-body strength exercise that works your chest, shoulders, and arms. They also engage your core for stabilization, making them a full-body workout.

Execution:

- Begin in a high plank position with your hands placed slightly wider than shoulder-width apart.
- Lower your body by bending your elbows while keeping your back straight.
- Push through your palms to return to the starting position.

Benefits: Push-ups are effective for building upper body strength, especially in the chest, shoulders, and triceps. They also improve core stability and can be modified to suit different fitness levels (e.g., knee push-ups for beginners).

4.Plank to push-up

Target area: Core, chest, shoulders, and arms.

This exercise combines the static hold of a plank with the dynamic movement of a push-up, giving your core and upper body a great workout.

Execution:

- Start in a forearm plank position, keeping your body in a straight line from head to heels.
- Push up onto your hands, one hand at a time, and move into a high plank.
- Lower back down onto your forearms, one arm at a time, to return to the starting position.
- Maintain a straight body line throughout the movement.

Benefits: The plank to push-up improves both core strength and upper body endurance. It requires stability and coordination, helping to engage multiple muscle groups simultaneously.

5.High knees

Target area: Core, legs (hip flexors), and cardiovascular system.

High knees are an effective cardio move that engages the core while also providing a full-body workout.

Execution:

- Stand with your feet hip-width apart.
- Drive your knees up toward your chest, alternating legs rapidly.
- Keep your arms bent at a 90-degree angle and pump them to match your knee movements.
- Focus on maintaining a quick pace while keeping your core engaged.

Benefits: High knees are an excellent cardiovascular exercise that increases heart rate, improves endurance, and strengthens your legs and core. This exercise also works on coordination and agility.

6.Mountain climbers

Target area: Full body, particularly the core, shoulders, and legs.

Mountain climbers are a dynamic move that combines cardio with strength training. They challenge your entire body, especially your core and upper body.

Execution:

- Start in a high plank position, keeping your hands directly under your shoulders.
- Bring one knee toward your chest, then quickly switch legs in a running motion, keeping your hips level.
- Focus on quick, controlled movements.

Benefits: Mountain climbers are great for building core strength, improving cardiovascular fitness, and engaging the shoulders and legs. This exercise also enhances coordination and endurance, making it a valuable addition to the 7-minute workout.

7.Lunges

Target area: Legs (quads, hamstrings, glutes), core.

Lunges are a fundamental lower-body exercise that works the legs and glutes while also improving balance and stability.

Execution:

- Stand with your feet hip-width apart.
- Step one leg forward and lower your body until both knees are bent at 90-degree angles.
- Push through the front foot to return to the starting position.
- Alternate legs for each repetition.

Benefits: Lunges are excellent for building strength in the lower body, improving balance, and enhancing flexibility in the hip flexors. They also engage the core for stabilization.

8.Tricep dips

Target area: Triceps, shoulders, and core.

Tricep dips are a fantastic way to target the triceps and build upper-body strength. This move can be performed using a chair or bench.

Execution:

- Sit on the edge of a bench or chair with your hands gripping the edge beside your hips.
- Slide your hips off the bench and lower your body by bending your elbows, keeping them close to your sides.
- Push through your palms to return to the starting position.

Benefits: Tricep dips are effective for strengthening the triceps and shoulders, helping to improve upper-body strength and tone the arms.

9.Burpees

Target area: Full body, particularly legs, chest, and core.

Burpees are one of the most challenging and effective full-body exercises, combining strength and cardio. They are great for building endurance and burning calories.

Execution:

- Start in a standing position.
- Drop into a squat and place your hands on the floor.
- Jump your feet back into a plank position.
- Perform a push-up, if desired.
- Jump your feet back toward your hands, then explosively jump into the air, reaching for the sky.
- Land softly and go straight into the next repetition.

Benefits: Burpees are a powerful move that engages nearly every muscle group in the body. They build strength, increase endurance, and significantly boost calorie burn.

10.Bicycle crunches

Target area: Core (abdominals and obliques).

Bicycle crunches target the core, specifically the abdominals and obliques, and help to improve core strength and definition.

Execution:

- Lie on your back with your hands behind your head and your knees bent.
- Lift your head, shoulders, and feet off the ground, bringing one knee toward your chest while extending the opposite leg.
- Twist your torso to bring your opposite elbow toward the bent knee, then switch sides in a pedaling motion.

Benefits: Bicycle crunches are excellent for toning the abdominal muscles and engaging the obliques, helping to sculpt and strengthen the core. They also improve coordination and flexibility.

11.Russian twists

Target area: Core (obliques, abs).

Russian twists focus on the obliques and help to build rotational strength, which is important for functional movement.

Execution:

- Sit on the floor with your knees bent and feet lifted off the ground.
- Lean back slightly to engage your core.
- Hold your hands together and rotate your torso from side to side, tapping the floor next to your hip each time.
- Keep the movement controlled and your core tight.

Benefits: Russian twists strengthen the obliques and core, improving stability and coordination. This exercise also aids in building endurance for rotational movements.

Conclusion

The 7-minute S.I.T. workout is designed to be a short yet highly effective routine that targets all areas of the body, combining strength training, cardiovascular exercise, and core work. The exercises included in this workout are carefully chosen to ensure that you engage multiple muscle groups, maximize calorie burn, and improve overall fitness in just seven minutes. Whether you're a beginner or an experienced fitness enthusiast, the 7-minute workout can be modified to meet your needs, making it a flexible and valuable addition to your routine.

Chapter 10: Safety and injury prevention

When it comes to any workout routine, especially a high-intensity interval training (HIIT) session like the 7-minute S.I.T. workout, safety should always be a top priority. The high intensity of these exercises can challenge both the body and the mind, but it also increases the risk of injury if not approached with caution. In this chapter, we'll explore the essential safety practices that can help you get the most out of your workout while minimizing the risk of injury.

1.The importance of proper warm-up

A proper warm-up is essential before engaging in any workout, but it becomes even more critical for high-intensity exercises like S.I.T. A warm-up helps prepare your muscles, joints, and cardiovascular system for the intense demands of the workout, reducing the risk of injury and improving your performance.

Why warm-up?

- **Increased blood flow:** A warm-up increases blood circulation to your muscles, making them more pliable and reducing the chance of strains.
- **Elevated heart rate:** By gradually raising your heart rate, you can avoid sudden spikes in intensity that could lead to dizziness or shortness of breath.
- **Joint mobility:** A dynamic warm-up can help improve flexibility and range of motion in your joints, lowering the risk of strains and sprains.

Recommended warm-up routine:

- **Dynamic stretches:** Focus on moving stretches that target the areas you will be using, such as leg swings, arm circles, and torso twists.

- **Light cardio:** Jogging in place or doing jumping jacks for 3-5 minutes can help get your heart rate up and blood flowing to your muscles.
- **Activation exercises:** Engage the muscles you'll be using in the workout. Bodyweight squats or lunges are great for warming up the lower body, while shoulder rolls or push-up holds can activate the upper body.

Taking the time to warm up will not only help you prevent injuries but will also improve your overall performance during the workout.

2.Focus on proper form

One of the most important elements of injury prevention is maintaining proper form throughout every exercise. When performing exercises like squats, push-ups, or lunges, incorrect form can lead to undue stress on your joints, muscles, and ligaments, increasing the risk of injuries like strains, sprains, or even more serious issues like torn muscles or ligaments.

Tips for maintaining proper form:

- **Start slow:** If you're new to the exercises in the S.I.T. workout, don't rush through them. Focus on performing each movement correctly at a slower pace before gradually increasing the speed and intensity.
- **Engage core muscles:** Always keep your core engaged to support your spine and maintain proper posture. This is especially important for exercises like planks, push-ups, and squats.
- **Alignment:** Pay attention to your body's alignment. For example, when performing squats, ensure your knees track over your toes and don't extend beyond them. In push-ups, make sure your hands are placed directly beneath your shoulders.
- **Breath control:** Proper breathing supports form and prevents unnecessary tension. Exhale as you exert force (e.g., when pushing up in a push-up), and inhale as you return to the starting position.

If you're unsure about your form, consider watching tutorial videos, working with a personal trainer, or using mirrors to check your alignment.

3.Progress gradually

One of the biggest mistakes people make when starting a new workout routine is pushing themselves too hard too quickly. While high-intensity training is great for results, it can also be demanding on your body. It's crucial to progress gradually, especially if you're new to fitness or have not been regularly exercising.

How to progress safely:

- **Start with modifications:** If you find certain exercises too difficult, don't hesitate to modify them. For example, if push-ups are too challenging, try knee push-ups until you build enough strength to perform full push-ups.

- **Increase intensity slowly:** Once you've mastered the basic form, you can start increasing the intensity of your workout by adding more repetitions or increasing the duration of each exercise.
- **Listen to your body:** If you feel any pain or discomfort during a workout, stop immediately. Pushing through pain can lead to more severe injuries. Mild soreness is normal, but sharp or persistent pain is a sign to rest or seek professional advice.

Gradual progression allows your body to adapt and build strength, reducing the likelihood of overexertion or injury.

4.Proper footwear and equipment

While the 7-minute S.I.T. workout is designed to be done without fancy equipment, there are a few essentials that will make your workout safer and more comfortable.

Footwear:

Proper shoes are crucial for providing the support and stability your body needs during high-intensity exercises. Wearing the wrong shoes can lead to foot, ankle, or knee injuries.

- **Supportive and comfortable shoes:** Choose shoes that offer good arch support and cushioning to absorb the impact of high-impact exercises like jumping jacks or burpees.
- **Non-slip soles:** Make sure your shoes have non-slip soles to help you maintain stability during exercises that require quick foot movements or changes in direction.

Surface:

Working out on a flat, stable surface is important for avoiding falls and maintaining proper form. If you're working out on a hard surface, consider using a yoga mat or an exercise mat to cushion your body during exercises that involve floor work.

5.Stay hydrated and rested

High-intensity workouts require energy, and maintaining hydration is crucial for keeping your performance at its best and preventing injury. Dehydration can lead to muscle cramps, dizziness, and a reduced ability to focus, all of which can increase the likelihood of injury.

Hydration tips:

- **Pre-workout hydration:** Drink water before you begin your workout to ensure that your body is well-hydrated.
- **During the workout:** Sip water throughout your workout, especially if you are sweating a lot. It's important to maintain hydration levels to keep your energy up.
- **Post-workout:** After the workout, continue drinking water to help with muscle recovery and to replenish any fluids lost through sweat.

Adequate rest and sleep are also critical for injury prevention. Overtraining or not allowing your muscles enough time to recover between workouts can increase the risk of injuries. Aim for 7-9 hours of sleep each night and include rest days in your weekly workout schedule.

6.Know your limits

While challenging yourself is important for progress, it's equally essential to know when to push and when to hold back. Everyone has a different fitness level, and what might be easy for one person could be difficult for another.

Signs you may be overdoing it:

- **Pain:** Pain is your body's way of telling you something is wrong. If you experience sharp pain during any exercise, stop immediately.
- **Dizziness or lightheadedness:** If you feel dizzy or lightheaded, take a break. These could be signs of dehydration, overexertion, or lack of proper nutrition.
- **Fatigue:** Feeling fatigued after a workout is normal, but if you are feeling overly exhausted or your body is failing to recover between sets, you may need to scale back the intensity or take more rest days.

It's essential to listen to your body and adjust your workouts accordingly. Overtraining can lead to injury, while recognizing your limits allows for safe progress.

7.Cool down and stretch

Just as a warm-up prepares your body for exercise, a cool-down is essential for helping your body recover afterward. Cooling down and stretching help prevent stiffness, reduce muscle soreness, and promote flexibility.

Cool-down routine:

- **Slow down gradually:** After your workout, reduce the intensity by walking around for a few minutes to bring your heart rate down slowly.
- **Stretching:** Focus on stretching the muscles you've worked during the session. Gentle stretches for the legs, arms, and back help reduce tightness and improve flexibility. Hold each stretch for at least 20-30 seconds without bouncing.

A proper cool-down routine helps facilitate muscle recovery and ensures that your body remains flexible and mobile.

Conclusion

Safety and injury prevention are key components of any successful workout routine, and the 7-minute S.I.T. workout is no exception. By following the guidelines outlined in this chapter—such as warming up properly, maintaining correct form, progressing gradually, and listening to your body—you can enjoy the benefits of high-intensity exercise without the risk of injury. Always remember that consistency, proper technique, and self-awareness are the cornerstones of safe and effective fitness practices.

Chapter 11: Warm-up for S.I.T.

Warming up before engaging in any workout is crucial, especially for high-intensity exercises like the 7-minute S.I.T. (Short Interval Training) workout. A proper warm-up prepares your body for the intense movements to come, increases your heart rate, and ensures that your muscles, joints, and nervous system are ready for action. In this chapter, we'll explore why a warm-up is so important, and provide you with an effective warm-up routine tailored for S.I.T. workouts.

1.Why is a warm-up important?

A warm-up is not just a "nice-to-have" element of a workout. It plays a vital role in preparing your body physically and mentally for the challenges ahead. The benefits of warming up include:

A.Preventing injuries

When you jump straight into intense exercises without warming up, your muscles, tendons, and ligaments are more prone to injury. A warm-up increases the elasticity of your muscles and improves joint mobility, reducing the risk of strains, sprains, or other injuries. The increased blood flow to your muscles helps them become more pliable, which is crucial when performing high-intensity exercises.

B.Increasing blood flow and heart rate

A proper warm-up gradually increases your heart rate, preparing your cardiovascular system for the demands of the workout. It also increases blood flow to your muscles, allowing them to perform better during the workout. A smooth transition into higher intensity ensures your body is ready to handle rapid movements and explosive exercises like burpees or jumping jacks.

C.Improving performance

When your muscles are adequately warmed up, they perform more efficiently. Warming up helps improve flexibility, mobility, and coordination. This can lead to better form during your workout and can help you get more out of your S.I.T. session, both in terms of performance and results.

D.Mental preparation

A warm-up not only prepares your body but also gets your mind focused. This mental preparation helps you enter the workout with the right mindset, reducing the chances of distractions and setting the tone for a productive session. It can also help reduce feelings of anxiety or hesitation, especially for beginners.

2.Types of warm-up

There are two main types of warm-up exercises: **dynamic warm-ups** and **static stretching**. For high-intensity workouts like S.I.T., dynamic warm-ups are more effective. Let's break down each type and understand their differences:

A.Dynamic warm-up

Dynamic warm-ups involve movement-based stretches that activate the muscles and increase blood flow. These exercises are designed to mimic the motions of the workout, making them perfect for preparing your body for the demands of high-intensity training. Dynamic movements improve your range of motion, enhance muscle activation, and help you avoid stiffness.

Common dynamic warm-up exercises include:

- **Leg swings** (forward-backward and side-to-side)
- **Arm circles** (small to large)
- **Torso twists**
- **Lunges with a twist**
- **High knees**
- **Butt kicks**

B.Static stretching

Static stretching involves holding a stretch for an extended period (typically 20-30 seconds) to improve flexibility. While static stretching is beneficial for improving overall flexibility, it's not ideal as part of a warm-up for intense workouts. In fact, static stretches before a workout can temporarily reduce muscle strength and power. For the S.I.T. workout, dynamic stretching is the preferred method to prepare your body for action.

3.Key areas to focus on during a warm-up

The warm-up should target the major muscle groups that will be engaged during the S.I.T. workout. By focusing on these areas, you ensure that your body is fully prepared for the exercises to come.

A.Lower body (Legs, Glutes, and Hips)

Since the 7-minute S.I.T. workout includes exercises like squats, lunges, and jumping jacks, your lower body will take the brunt of the work. Warming up the legs, glutes, and hips is crucial for injury prevention and optimal performance.

Dynamic warm-up exercises for lower body:

- **Leg swings:** Swing your legs forward and backward to loosen the hips and activate the hamstrings, quadriceps, and glutes.
- **Lunges with a twist:** Step forward into a lunge and twist your torso to engage the core and improve hip flexibility.
- **Hip circles:** Stand with your hands on your hips and make large circles with your hips to loosen the hip joint.
- **High knees:** Jog in place while bringing your knees up toward your chest. This engages the hip flexors and warms up the legs.
- **Butt kicks:** While jogging in place, kick your heels up towards your glutes to activate the hamstrings and improve hip mobility.

B.Upper body (Arms, Shoulders, and Chest)

The S.I.T. workout also incorporates upper-body exercises such as push-ups, tricep dips, and planks. Warming up the arms, shoulders, and chest helps ensure that your upper body can handle these movements without strain.

Dynamic warm-up exercises for upper body:

- **Arm circles:** Stand with your arms extended and make circles, starting small and gradually increasing the size. This will warm up the shoulders and arms.
- **Torso twists:** Stand with your feet shoulder-width apart and twist your torso from side to side to warm up the upper back and shoulders.
- **Shoulder rolls:** Roll your shoulders forward and backward to loosen the shoulder joints.
- **Arm swings:** Swing your arms forward and backward, crossing them over your chest to activate the shoulders, arms, and chest.

C.Core (Abdominals and Lower Back)

The core plays an essential role in stabilizing your body during many of the S.I.T. exercises, including planks, push-ups, and squats. A warm-up that activates the core muscles will help improve stability and overall performance.

Dynamic warm-up exercises for core:

- **Torso twists (again):** These not only warm up the upper body but also engage the obliques and abs.
- **Standing side crunches:** Stand with your hands behind your head and bring your knee up toward your elbow, alternating sides to engage the obliques and lower abs.

- **Cat-cow stretch:** On all fours, arch your back toward the ceiling and then dip it toward the floor, alternating between flexion and extension to mobilize the spine and activate the core.
- **Plank walkouts:** Stand up straight, bend at the waist, and walk your hands out into a plank position. This warms up the core, chest, shoulders, and hips.

4.Full warm-Up routine for S.I.T.

Now that we've covered the theory behind warming up and the key muscle groups to target, let's put it all together into a simple but effective warm-up routine for the 7-minute S.I.T. workout.

Step-by-step routine:

1.**March or jog in place (1 minute):** Start by gently marching or jogging in place. This helps gradually increase your heart rate and get your blood flowing to all areas of the body.

2.**Leg swings (30 seconds per leg):** Hold onto a wall or chair for balance and swing one leg forward and backward, gradually increasing the range of motion. Switch legs after 30 seconds.

3.**Arm circles (1 minute):** Extend your arms out to the sides and make circles, starting small and gradually making them larger. Alternate directions after 30 seconds.

4.**Lunges with a twist (1 minute):** Step forward into a lunge, twist your torso toward the side of your front leg, and return to the standing position. Alternate legs as you go.

5.**Torso twists (1 minute):** Stand with your feet shoulder-width apart and rotate your torso side to side, keeping your hips stable. This helps activate the core and upper body.

6.**High knees (1 minute):** Jog in place while driving your knees up toward your chest. Keep your posture upright and engage your core.

7.**Butt kicks (1 minute):** While jogging in place, kick your heels up toward your glutes to engage your hamstrings and activate your lower body.

8.**Plank walkouts (1 minute):** Stand tall, then bend at the waist and walk your hands forward into a plank position. Hold for a few seconds, then walk your hands back toward your feet and stand up.

By the end of this warm-up routine, your body will be fully prepared for the intense movements in the S.I.T. workout. Your heart rate will be elevated, your muscles will be activated, and your joints will be primed for movement.

---

5. Conclusion

A proper warm-up is a crucial part of any high-intensity workout, especially one as demanding as the 7-minute S.I.T. workout. Taking the time to prepare your body through dynamic stretches and activation exercises will not only reduce the risk of injury but also enhance your performance during the workout. Remember to warm up consistently before each session to get the most out of your training and stay safe. With the right warm-up, you'll be ready to crush your S.I.T. workout and enjoy the benefits of improved strength, endurance, and overall fitness.

Chapter 12: The classic S.I.T. workout

The classic S.I.T. (Short Interval Training) workout is a powerful and effective way to improve cardiovascular fitness, build strength, and burn fat in a short amount of time. This high-intensity, seven-minute workout includes a combination of bodyweight exercises designed to push your body to its limits while minimizing the time commitment. In this chapter, we will explore the structure of the classic S.I.T. workout, the exercises it includes, and how to execute it properly for maximum results.

1.The structure of the classic S.I.T. workout

The classic S.I.T. workout follows a simple structure: seven minutes of intense, full-body exercises with minimal rest in between. The goal of this workout is to maximize intensity within a short time frame to push your body into a state of "fat-burning" afterburn. These seven minutes are broken down into 30-second intervals of intense exercise followed by a 10-second rest. Each exercise in the routine is chosen to challenge different muscle groups while keeping the heart rate elevated.

A.High intensity, short duration

The key to the effectiveness of the classic S.I.T. workout is the combination of high-intensity exercise and brief rest periods. By pushing your body to work as hard as possible for short bursts of time, you can maximize calorie burn and stimulate muscle growth in a very efficient manner. This method helps improve both aerobic and anaerobic fitness, making it an ideal workout for people with limited time.

B.Rest intervals

The 10-second rest period between exercises is designed to allow just enough recovery to maintain high intensity without allowing your heart rate to drop too much. During the rest period, you can focus on taking deep breaths to recover and prepare for the next exercise. Although 10 seconds may seem short, it is typically enough to catch your breath and get ready for the next burst of energy.

2.Exercises in the classic S.I.T. workout

The classic S.I.T. workout consists of seven bodyweight exercises, each targeting different muscle groups to create a balanced full-body workout. These exercises are chosen for their ability to engage multiple muscle groups simultaneously, making them highly effective for fat loss, muscle toning, and strength building.

A. Jumping Jacks (30 seconds)

Jumping jacks are a great exercise to get your heart rate up quickly. This full-body movement engages the arms, legs, and core while improving cardiovascular endurance. By including jumping jacks in the S.I.T. workout, you start with a fast-paced, high-intensity exercise that activates your entire body and prepares you for the intensity to come.

How to do jumping jacks:

- Stand with your feet together and arms by your sides.
- Jump your feet out wide while raising your arms overhead.
- Jump back to the starting position with your feet together and arms by your sides.
- Repeat for 30 seconds, keeping the movement fluid and controlled.

B. Wall Sit (30 seconds)

Wall sits are an isometric exercise that targets the lower body, particularly the quadriceps, glutes, and hamstrings. This exercise forces you to hold a seated position against a wall, which challenges your endurance and strength.

How to do a wall sit:

- Stand with your back against a wall and feet about hip-width apart.
- Slide down the wall until your knees are bent at a 90-degree angle, as if you were sitting in an invisible chair.
- Hold the position for 30 seconds, keeping your back flat against the wall and your knees in line with your toes.

C.Push-ups (30 seconds)

Push-ups are a classic bodyweight exercise that targets the chest, shoulders, and triceps, while also engaging the core and lower body for stability. They are an essential part of the classic S.I.T. workout because they provide both upper body strength training and core activation.

How to do push-ups:

- Start in a plank position with your hands placed directly under your shoulders.
- Lower your body down by bending your elbows, keeping your body in a straight line from head to heels.
- Push yourself back up to the starting position.
- Repeat for 30 seconds, focusing on maintaining proper form and controlled movements.

D.Squats (30 seconds)

Squats are a foundational lower-body exercise that primarily targets the quadriceps, glutes, and hamstrings. In the classic S.I.T. workout, squats help build strength and endurance in the legs and improve overall lower body stability.

How to do squats:

- Stand with your feet shoulder-width apart, with your toes slightly pointed outward.
- Bend your knees and lower your hips as if you were sitting back into a chair.
- Keep your chest up and your knees behind your toes as you squat down.
- Push through your heels to stand back up, returning to the starting position.
- Repeat for 30 seconds, focusing on depth and form.

E.Plank (30 seconds)

The plank is a core exercise that targets the abdominals, lower back, and shoulders. It is an isometric exercise that helps build core strength and stability, which is important for maintaining proper posture and alignment during other exercises.

How to do a plank:

- Start in a forearm plank position with your elbows directly beneath your shoulders and your body in a straight line from head to heels.
- Engage your core, glutes, and legs to keep your body stable and avoid sagging in the lower back.
- Hold the position for 30 seconds, breathing steadily and maintaining proper alignment.

F.High knees (30 seconds)

High knees are a cardio exercise that also targets the hip flexors, quads, and core. This exercise increases heart rate and promotes coordination, making it an excellent choice for the S.I.T. workout's high-intensity intervals.

How to do high knees:

- Stand tall with your feet hip-width apart.

- Jog in place while driving your knees up toward your chest, alternating legs as quickly as possible.
- Engage your core and pump your arms to increase the intensity.
- Continue for 30 seconds, maintaining a quick pace.

G.Burpees (30 seconds)

Burpees are one of the most intense and challenging exercises included in the classic S.I.T. workout. This full-body exercise targets the legs, core, chest, and shoulders, making it a great way to finish off the workout with an explosive movement that burns calories and builds strength.

How to do burpees:

- Start standing with your feet shoulder-width apart.
- Squat down and place your hands on the floor, then jump your feet back into a plank position.
- Perform a push-up (optional), then jump your feet back toward your hands.
- Explode upward, jumping into the air with your arms extended overhead.
- Land softly and repeat for 30 seconds.

3.How to perform the classic S.I.T. workout

Now that you understand the individual exercises in the classic S.I.T. workout, it's time to put them all together into a cohesive workout routine. The workout consists of seven exercises, each performed for 30 seconds, followed by 10 seconds of rest. Complete one round of the full workout, and then you can repeat the circuit if you have time and energy to do so.

The classic S.I.T. workout routine:

1.Jumping jacks (30 seconds)

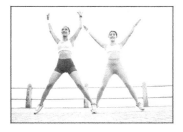

2.Wall sit (30 seconds)

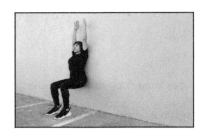

3.Push-ups (30 seconds)

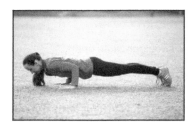

4.Squats (30 seconds)

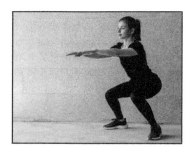

5.Plank (30 seconds)

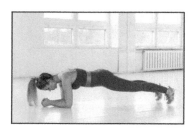

6.High knees (30 seconds)

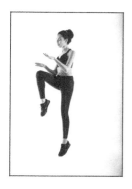

7.Burpees (30 seconds)

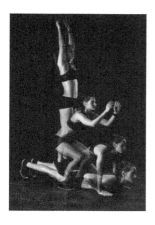

Rest for 10 seconds after each exercise, and perform the entire circuit without stopping. If you're able to, repeat the circuit for a total of 2-3 rounds for an even more intense workout. Always listen to your body, and take additional rest if needed.

4.Modifications for beginners

While the classic S.I.T. workout is designed to be challenging, it can be modified to suit different fitness levels. For beginners or those who may not be able to perform some of the exercises at full intensity, here are a few modifications:

- **Wall sit:** Reduce the time or perform the exercise for shorter intervals if holding the position for 30 seconds is too difficult.
- **Push-ups:** Start with knee push-ups or incline push-ups (with your hands on a raised surface) to reduce the difficulty.
- **Burpees:** Perform half-burpees by omitting the push-up and jumping, focusing only on the squat and plank portion.

5.Conclusion

An excellent and efficient method to increase strength, endurance, and cardiovascular fitness in only seven minutes is the original S.I.T. workout. This workout is great for getting a full-body workout quickly since it uses a range of exercises that target various muscle groups. Whether you're just starting out or have been working out for a while, the S.I.T. workout can be customized to suit your fitness level, making it a great choice for anyone looking to get fit and burn fat quickly.

Chapter 13: Variations of the 7-minute workout

There is no short and successful fitness regimen that does not include the 7-minute workout. People who lead hectic lives but still want to be physically active but don't have time for lengthy workouts could benefit from its efficiency, adaptability, and lack of complexity. While the original 7-minute exercise is great for overall fitness, there are a number of adaptations you may try to reach more specific fitness objectives, avoid training plateaus, and spice up your routine. Various 7-minute workout plans targeting various aspects of fitness, such as strength training, cardiovascular health, flexibility, or weight loss, will be covered in this chapter.

1.Strength-focused 7-minute workout

While the classic 7-minute workout does include strength-building exercises like push-ups and squats, a variation can be designed specifically to emphasize strength. This variation includes exercises that challenge different muscle groups and are designed to improve muscle tone and overall strength.

Structure:

Legs, chest, backwards, shoulder blades, and arms are the primary targets of this variant's workouts. The goal of this workout is to increase strength and endurance via the use of bodyweight movements. For example, squats, lunges, push-ups, and tricep dips can be included for an overall strength boost.

Example:

    1.Push-ups (30 seconds)

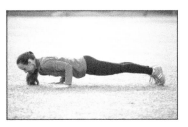

    2.Squats (30 seconds)

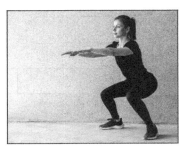

    3.Plank (30 seconds)

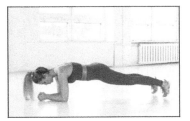

4.Tricep dips (30 seconds)

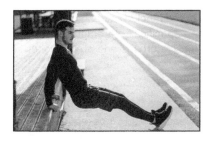

5.Lunge jumps (30 seconds)

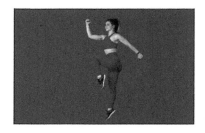

6.Wall sit (30 seconds)

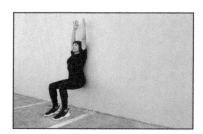

7.Superman hold (30 seconds)

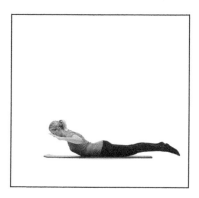

This workout builds muscle by utilizing multi-joint movements, which engage various muscle groups simultaneously. By focusing on strength, this variation helps you build muscle endurance and adds a more targeted approach to the typical 7-minute workout.

2.Cardio-focused 7-minute workout

A cardio-focused variation of the 7-minute workout places an emphasis on heart-pumping exercises designed to improve cardiovascular health, stamina, and fat burning. These exercises incorporate higher-intensity moves that keep your heart rate elevated, leading to greater calorie burn and enhanced aerobic capacity.

Structure:

Cardio-focused exercises include movements such as jumping jacks, high knees, burpees, and mountain climbers. These exercises get your heart rate up quickly and can help you improve your endurance over time. To maximize calorie burn, aim for movements that involve multiple muscle groups and promote fast transitions between exercises.

Example:

1.Jumping jacks (30 seconds)

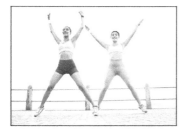

2.Burpees (30 seconds)

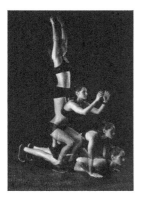

3.High knees (30 seconds)

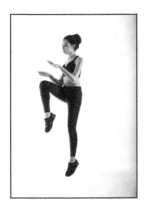

4.Mountain climbers (30 seconds)

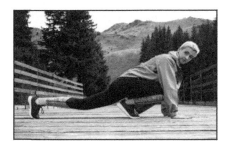

5.Jump squats (30 seconds)

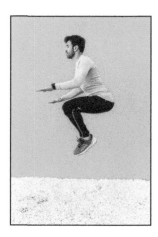

6.Skater jumps (30 seconds)

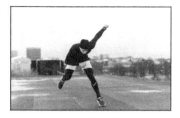

7.Fast feet (30 seconds)

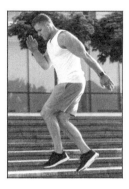

The goal of this workout variation is to keep your body in a continuous state of motion, helping to elevate your heart rate and improve cardiovascular health. This workout is perfect for those looking to improve stamina, burn fat, and increase overall endurance.

3.Flexibility and mobility-focused 7-minute workout

Flexibility and mobility are often overlooked in many workout routines. A flexibility and mobility-focused variation of the 7-minute workout aims to improve the range of motion, reduce the risk of injury, and increase muscle elasticity. These exercises focus on dynamic stretches, mobility drills, and flexibility-enhancing movements.

Structure:

This version includes exercises such as dynamic stretches, hip openers, and movements that improve joint mobility. The idea is to focus on improving flexibility through movement rather than static stretching alone.

Example:

1.Arm circles (30 seconds)

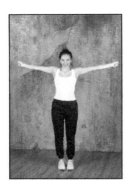

2. Hip circles (30 seconds)

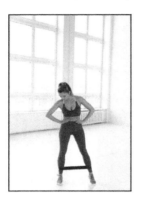

3. Lunge with a twist (30 seconds)

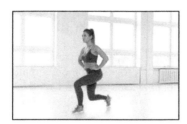

4. Downward dog to cobra flow (30 seconds)

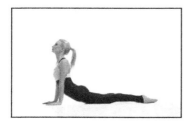

5.Standing side stretch (30 seconds)

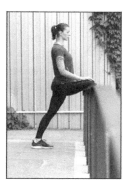

6.Leg swings (30 seconds)

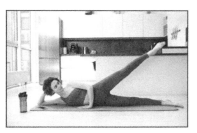

7.Cat-cow stretch (30 seconds)

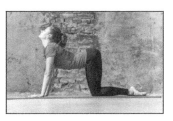

In this workout, the exercises emphasize active flexibility, which helps you move more fluidly and reduces muscle tightness. It also prepares your body for more intense exercise, increasing the range of motion and joint mobility.

4.Core-focused 7-minute workout

A core-focused variation targets the muscles of the abdominal region, lower back, and obliques. A strong core is essential for overall fitness, as it plays a crucial role in maintaining stability, balance, and proper posture. This variation emphasizes core-strengthening exercises that work all aspects of the core.

Structure:

In this variation, each exercise is designed to engage different parts of the core. The exercises will challenge the abdominal muscles, lower back, and obliques, helping to build a strong, stable core.

Example:

    1.Plank (30 seconds)

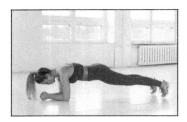

    2.Russian twists (30 seconds)

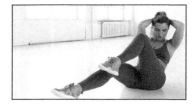

    3.Bicycle crunches (30 seconds)

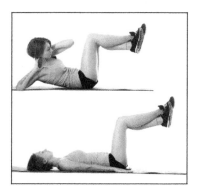

4.Leg raises (30 seconds)

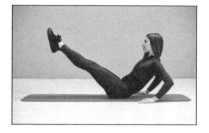

5.Side plank (30 seconds each side)

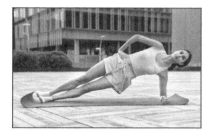

6.Mountain climbers (30 seconds)

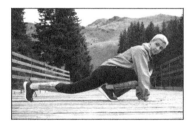

7.Flutter kicks (30 seconds)

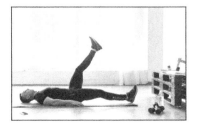

By engaging the entire core, this workout helps improve overall abdominal strength and stability. It's ideal for those looking to build a strong core and improve posture.

5.Low-impact 7-minute workout

A low-impact variation of the 7-minute workout is perfect for individuals with joint pain, beginners, or anyone who prefers less intense movements. This workout eliminates high-impact exercises like burpees and jumping jacks and focuses on movements that are gentler on the joints, while still providing an effective workout.

Structure:

The low-impact variation includes exercises like step-touch, slow squats, and modified lunges. These movements keep your heart rate elevated without the harsh impact on the joints that can be problematic for some people.

Example:

1.March in place (30 seconds)

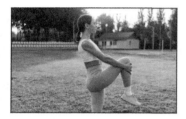

2.Step-touch (30 seconds)

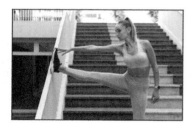

3.Wall push-ups (30 seconds)

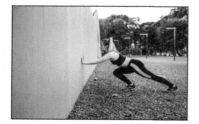

4.Slow squats (30 seconds)

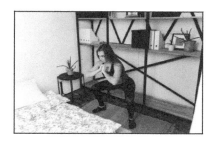

5.Seated leg raises (30 seconds)

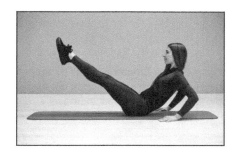

6.Standing oblique crunches (30 seconds)

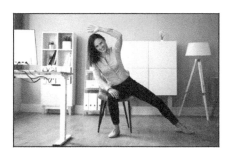

7.Heel raises (30 seconds)

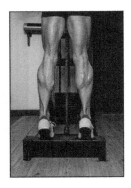

This variation is great for those who want to get the benefits of a full-body workout without putting excess strain on their knees, hips, or back. It's a more accessible alternative that still challenges the body and increases fitness.

6.Total body 7-minute workout

The total body variation of the 7-minute workout combines elements of strength, cardio, and core work into one comprehensive session. This version is designed to target all major muscle groups, providing a balanced, full-body workout that helps increase strength, burn fat, and improve cardiovascular health.

Structure:

The total body workout includes a variety of exercises to target different muscle groups, ensuring that no part of the body is neglected. Each exercise engages multiple muscle groups simultaneously, making it a time-efficient way to get a complete workout.

Example:

1.Jumping jacks (30 seconds)

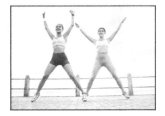

2.Push-ups (30 seconds)

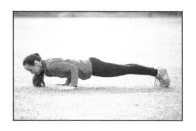

3.Squats (30 seconds)

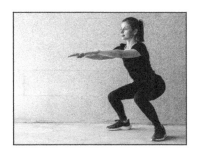

4.Plank (30 seconds)

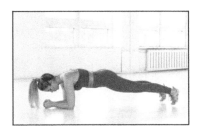

5.High knees (30 seconds)

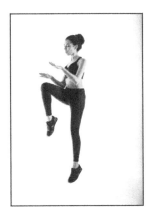

6.Burpees (30 seconds)

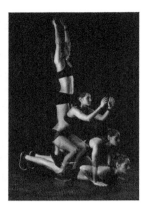

7.Superman hold (30 seconds)

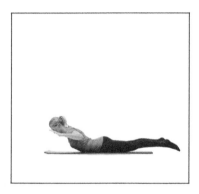

This full-body workout is perfect for those who want an all-around, time-efficient routine. By combining strength, endurance, and flexibility exercises, this variation is effective for improving overall fitness and toning muscles.

7.Advanced 7-minute workout

For more experienced fitness enthusiasts looking for a greater challenge, the advanced 7-minute workout pushes your limits with more intense and complex movements. This variation often incorporates exercises that require greater coordination, strength, and power.

Structure:

The advanced workout includes exercises like jump lunges, squat thrusts, and explosive push-ups. These movements are designed to challenge the body and increase muscular strength, coordination, and endurance. The intensity is higher, and the rest periods may be slightly shortened.

Example:

1.Jump lunges (30 seconds)

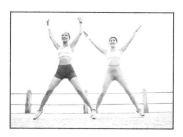

2.Push-ups (30 seconds)

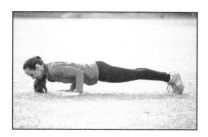

3.Jump squats (30 seconds)

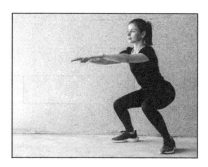

4.Plank with shoulder taps (30 seconds)

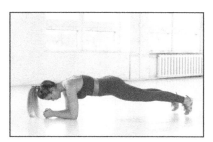

5.Burpee to push-up (30 seconds)

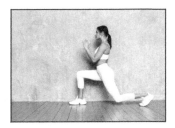

6.Tuck jumps (30 seconds)

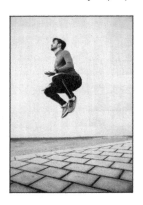

7.Mountain climbers (30 seconds)

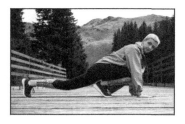

This variation is for those who are already in good shape and are looking for an advanced challenge. It incorporates explosive movements to enhance power and agility while still keeping the workout within the 7-minute window.

8.Conclusion

The 7-minute workout is versatile enough to accommodate a wide range of fitness levels and goals. Whether you're looking to build strength, increase cardiovascular endurance, improve flexibility, or target specific muscle groups, there is a variation of the 7-minute workout that suits your needs. The key to staying motivated and avoiding workout plateaus is to mix things up regularly. By exploring different variations, you can keep your workouts fresh, engaging, and effective.

Chapter 14: The role of nutrition and hydration

Exercise is just one component of a healthy lifestyle that contributes to overall fitness and well-being. Proper diet and hydration greatly boost the results of the 7-minute workout (S.I.T.), which gives a strong burst of activity that enhances cardiovascular health, strength, and endurance. Regardless of your fitness objective—weight loss, muscle gain, or general health—the food and drink you consume prior to, during, and following exercise can have a profound impact. In this section, we will delve into the importance of staying hydrated and eating well for a S.I.T. workout. By fuelling your body correctly, you may reach your fitness objectives much more quickly.

1.Nutrition: Fueling your workout

Nutrition is fundamental to the success of any fitness program, including the 7-minute workout. In order to train effectively, recuperate properly, and gain muscle over time, your body requires the energy that comes from the food you eat. The function of carbs, proteins, and fats, the three main macronutrients, in sustaining an efficient exercise program will be covered in this section.

A.Carbohydrates: The body's primary energy source

When you're doing out at a high intensity, such in the S.I.T. routine, your body uses carbohydrates for energy. Your muscles & brain get their fuel from glucose, which is made when you eat carbohydrates. In high-intensity workouts, such as those that involve short bursts of energy, carbohydrates play a vital role in maintaining your performance. Without adequate carbohydrate intake, your energy levels may deplete quickly, leading to early fatigue and reduced workout efficiency.

There are two types of carbohydrates: simple and complex.

- **Simple carbs**: These are quickly digested and absorbed into the bloodstream, providing fast energy. Foods like fruit, honey, and certain types of sugary snacks are examples of simple carbs. While these can be helpful for a quick energy boost, they should be consumed in moderation, especially if you're aiming to lose weight.
- **Complex carbs**: Their gradual breakdown ensures a continuous flow of energy. Complex carbs are abundant in foods including beans, vegetables, and whole grains (such as quinoa, oats, and brown rice). You can keep going strong during your workout if you include these in your before-workout breakfast.

B.Protein: Building and repairing muscle

Protein is essential for muscle repair and growth. When you engage in exercises like the 7-minute workout, your muscles undergo microtears, which need to be repaired to get stronger. Protein helps rebuild these muscles, making it a vital component of your post-workout nutrition.

For those engaging in regular exercise, including resistance training and high-intensity workouts, protein should be consumed both before and after workouts. Choose protein-rich foods that are easy on the digestive system, such chicken, turkey, eggs, fish, or legumes, beans, and tofu.

Twenty to thirty grammes of protein is the sweet spot for post-workout muscle repair and recovery, so that's what most people do. To get the most out of your muscles' recuperation time after exercise, eat some protein within half an hour to an hour.

C.Healthy fats: Supporting long-term energy

While fats often get a bad reputation, they are crucial for long-term energy and overall health. Healthy fats support various body functions, including hormone production, joint health, and nutrient absorption. Additionally, fats can provide a more sustained form of energy during low-intensity or longer-duration activities.

Sources of healthy fats include:

- Avocados
- Nuts and seeds
- Olive oil
- Fatty fish (like salmon and mackerel)

Incorporating moderate amounts of healthy fats into your diet, especially in post-workout meals, can help keep your energy levels balanced throughout the day.

2.Hydration: The essential element for performance and recovery

Proper hydration is essential for any workout, including the 7-minute workout. Our bodies are made up of approximately 60% water, and hydration plays a key role in nearly every physiological function, including muscle function, temperature regulation, and nutrient transport. Dehydration, even in mild forms, can significantly impact your performance during workouts, leaving you feeling fatigued, sluggish, and weak.

A. The importance of hydration during the S.I.T. workout

During high-intensity workouts like S.I.T., your body loses water through sweat. This fluid loss needs to be replaced to prevent dehydration, which can affect your strength, stamina, and overall performance. When you're dehydrated, your muscles do not perform at their full potential, and your ability to recover post-workout is impaired.

It's recommended to drink water before, during, and after your workout. If you're working out intensely for 7 minutes or longer, aim to sip water throughout your session. A good guideline is to drink about 7 to 10 ounces of water every 20 minutes during your workout, depending on your sweat rate and the workout's intensity.

B. Electrolyte balance: Replenishing sodium, potassium, and magnesium

In addition to water, it's also important to replenish electrolytes—minerals like sodium, potassium, and magnesium that help regulate muscle function, fluid balance, and nerve signaling. When you sweat, you lose electrolytes, which can lead to cramping, fatigue, and even dizziness if not replenished.

For shorter, less intense workouts like the 7-minute S.I.T. session, plain water is usually sufficient. However, for more intense or extended workouts, or if you sweat a lot, you may want to consume beverages that contain electrolytes. Natural sources like coconut water, or sports drinks that are low in sugar, can be beneficial for restoring electrolyte balance.

C. Pre-workout hydration

Before beginning your S.I.T. workout, aim to hydrate at least 30 minutes to an hour in advance. Drinking water beforehand ensures that your body is properly fueled and ready to perform. Dehydration can result in early fatigue, reduced endurance, and a decreased ability to focus.

A good pre-workout hydration strategy is to drink about 8 to 16 ounces of water, depending on your body size and how much you've been drinking throughout the day. This will allow your body to maintain optimal fluid levels for the workout ahead.

3. Timing of meals: Pre- and post-workout nutrition

What you eat before and after your workout is just as important as the nutrition you consume throughout the day. Proper meal timing helps optimize performance, recovery, and muscle growth.

A. Pre-workout nutrition

Giving your body the fuel it needs to function at its peak is the main objective of pre-workout nutrition. To prepare your body for exercise, eat a healthy meal at least an hour or two before you hit the gym. The ideal components of this meal include carbs for fuel, protein for building muscle, and a modest quantity of healthy fats.

Example of a pre-workout meal:

- Banana slices, almond butter, and whole grain bread

- Greek yoghurt topped with oats and berries

- Blended spinach, oats, almond milk, and protein powder into a delicious smoothie.

A protein bar, a handful of almonds or a banana eaten 30 minutes before exercise might be just as effective as a complete meal if you're short on time.

B. Nutrition after exercise

Restoring energy storage and aiding muscle recovery are two of the most critical things to do after a workout. Between between thirty and sixty minutes after your activity, it's best to have a snack or a meal that has carbs and protein. This aids in the regeneration of muscle tissue (protein) and the restoration of glycogen (carbohydrates).

Example of a post-workout meal:

- Quinoa and grilled chicken served with steamed veggies
- A protein-packed smoothie made with almond milk, spinach, fruit, and powdered protein.
- A whole grain wrap with turkey, avocado, and mixed greens

Post-workout nutrition supports muscle recovery, reduces soreness, and helps your body adapt and grow stronger from the workout.

4.The role of supplements in nutrition

Some people choose to take supplements to aid in their fitness objectives, even though a healthy diet may supply most of the vitamins and minerals your body requires. But a healthy diet is still the most important thing, and supplements aren't meant to take the place of it. Supplements like these are ubiquitous, and they could help those who perform intense workouts:

- **Protein powder**: If you have trouble getting enough protein from dietary sources, this might help with muscle healing and repair.

- Because it gives muscles more energy, creatine may help athletes perform better during high-intensity workouts.

- Branched-chain amino acids, or BCAAs, can help with muscle repair and pain.

- Taking a multivitamin can help you get all the nutrients you need each day, which is particularly important if you have food limitations.

Because each person's nutritional needs are unique, it's important to talk to a doctor or nutritionist before starting a supplement regimen.

5.Conclusion

Nutrition and hydration play a pivotal role in your ability to perform well during your 7-minute workout and recover afterward.You may enhance your performance, development of muscle, and general health by providing the body with the correct nutrients and maintaining an adequate water intake. Keep in mind that working out is just half the battle; your nutrition also plays a major role in determining how quickly you reach your fitness objectives.

Chapter 15: Progression and increasing intensity

When it comes to fitness, one of the keys to achieving long-term success is progression. Whether you're new to the S.I.T. workout or you've been incorporating it into your routine for a while, it's important to continually challenge your body in order to improve your fitness level. Progression doesn't always mean doing more, faster, or harder right away, but rather making intentional adjustments over time to keep your body adapting and improving. In this chapter, we will explore the principles of progression, how to safely and effectively increase intensity in your 7-minute S.I.T. workout, and how to track and measure your progress.

1.Understanding progression in fitness

Progression is the gradual increase in the intensity, volume, or difficulty of a workout over time. It's based on the principle of overloading your muscles and cardiovascular system in a way that pushes them to adapt. As you continue to challenge your body, your muscles get stronger, your endurance improves, and your overall fitness level rises. Without progression, your body can hit a plateau, where improvements in strength, endurance, or performance stagnate.

Progression can take many forms, and it's important to focus on a balanced approach to prevent injury, burnout, or frustration. There are several ways to introduce progression into your 7-minute workout routine, and in this chapter, we will discuss different methods that you can apply to increase the intensity and effectiveness of your workouts.

2.Methods of progression

What works best for you in terms of intensity and results during your S.I.T. workout will vary from person to person based on factors including personal preference, present fitness level, and desired outcomes. If you want to get the most of your 7-minute exercise, try these strategies:

A.Increasing duration or time

The simplest way to progress in your 7-minute workout is by extending the duration of each exercise or the entire workout itself. While the classic S.I.T. workout is structured for 7 minutes, you can challenge yourself by adding more time. You can do this by either increasing the length of each exercise to 45 seconds or 1 minute, or by adding an additional round to the circuit.

For example:

- **Start with 7 minutes**: Every exercise should be done for 30 seconds, with a 10-second break in between.

- Workout for 40 seconds straight with just five seconds of break in between (Progression 1).

- The second progression calls for doing each exercise for a full minute without stopping.

- Thirdly, extend the workout to a total of fourteen minutes by including one extra circuit.

This method of increasing the duration allows you to gradually build stamina, pushing yourself further while giving your body time to adapt.

B.Increasing intensity by adding variations

Another great way to increase intensity is by changing up the exercises to make them more challenging. Instead of performing basic exercises like regular squats or push-ups, you can modify them to involve more muscle groups, increase the range of motion, or add explosive movements.

Here are some examples of how you can modify common S.I.T. exercises:

- **Push-ups → Plyometric push-ups** (where you push off the ground with enough force to momentarily lift your hands off the ground)
- **Squats → Jump squats** (a squat followed by an explosive jump)
- **Lunges → Jump lunges** (performing a lunge and then jumping to switch legs mid-air)
- **Plank → Plank to push-up** (transitioning from a forearm plank to a high plank and back down)

By increasing the difficulty of each exercise, you challenge your muscles in different ways, leading to more effective strength and endurance gains.

C.Reducing rest time

You may also increase the intensity of the workout by decreasing the amount of time you rest between sets or circuits. Your cardiovascular system needs to work harder to keep up with your activity level if you don't rest enough. You may increase your endurance and fat-burning capacity by keeping your heart rate raised during shorter rest times. This forces your body to work harder to recover.

For example:

- **Classic S.I.T. workout**: 30 seconds per exercise, 10 seconds of rest between exercises.
- **Progression 1**: 30 seconds of workout with a 5-second break in between.
- Step 2: Perform each exercise for 30 seconds without resting in between.

By limiting recovery time, you create a more intense workout, which challenges your cardiovascular system and accelerates calorie burning.

D.Adding resistance

Including external resistance in your S.I.T. routine will help you get to the next level. An effective strategy to enhance muscular growth and strength is to use resistance bands, weighted vests, or dumbbells to raise the strain on your muscles. Squats, squats push-ups, and planks become more challenging and provide new physical obstacles when you incorporate resistance into your workout routine.

For example:

- **Push-ups**: To make the push-up more challenging, try wearing a vest with weights or wrapping a resistance band across your back.
- **Squats**: Hold dumbbells or a kettlebell while performing squats to engage more muscle groups and increase the intensity.
- **Lunges**: Hold a pair of dumbbells at your sides to intensify the movement and challenge your lower body more.

By adding resistance, you stimulate muscle growth and increase the challenge of your S.I.T. workout.

3.Measuring progress and tracking results

If you want to stay motivated and make sure you reach your fitness objectives, tracking how you're doing is key. By maintaining a record of your exercises, you may observe observable growth over time and pinpoint areas that require more effort. You may track your development in several ways.

A.Keep a workout journal

A workout journal allows you to record the details of each session, including the exercises performed, the duration, rest time, and any modifications made. This helps you see how you're progressing over time. For example, if you started with 30-second intervals for each exercise, you might notice after a few weeks that you're now able to perform each exercise for 45 seconds with less rest between movements.

B.Track performance and strength gains

Tracking your performance is an excellent way to measure your progress. For example, keep track of how many push-ups or squats you can do in 30 seconds. If you're able to complete more repetitions over time, it's a sign that you're gaining strength and endurance. By using this metric to monitor your progress, you can find out where you're excelling and where you still have room to grow.

C. Make use of fitness-related applications or wearables

Utilising fitness applications or wearable gadgets that track vital signs, calorie expenditure, and other performance indicators is something that many individuals find useful. These aids can show you how your organism is reacting to the higher intensity and how far you've come as a whole.

4.Avoiding plateaus: Keeping your workouts fresh

Over time, as your body adapts to a workout, you may hit a plateau where your progress slows or stops. To continue improving, you need to make adjustments to your workouts regularly. If you find that you're no longer seeing the same level of improvement, it's time to shake up your routine. Here are some strategies to avoid plateaus:

- **Change exercises**: Introduce new exercises to your S.I.T. workout that target different muscle groups or work muscles in a different way.
- **Switch up intensity**: Gradually increase the difficulty by combining different progression methods—add resistance, shorten rest times, or increase the duration of exercises.
- **Periodization**: Using periodisation, you may train in cycles of different intensities, such as strength, endurance, and power for a certain period of time before moving on to something else.

By constantly challenging yourself and making strategic adjustments, you can continue progressing and avoid getting stuck in a plateau.

5.Conclusion

A important component of any fitness regimen is progression, which allows for continuous increases over time. Improving your outcomes from your 7-minute S.I.T. exercise is as simple as gradually pushing yourself to your limitations, whether that's in terms of intensity, time, or complexity. Make sure you keep making progress towards your fitness objectives by tracking your progress, monitoring your performance, and adjusting your routines accordingly. The long-term advantages of the S.I.T. exercise may be yours if you're patient, consistent, and dedicated to improving your fitness level gradually.

Chapter 16: Training without equipment

One of the major appeals of the 7-minute S.I.T. workout is its simplicity and accessibility. It requires no special equipment, making it ideal for people who want to get fit but don't have access to a gym or expensive workout gear. Among the several advantages of training without equipment are its portability, low cost, and the freedom to work out whenever and wherever you choose. Adapting the 7-minute S.I.T. fitness to be completely equipment-free is one of the topics we'll cover in this chapter, along with other strategies for making the most of a workout regimen that doesn't use any machines or tools.

1.The power of bodyweight training

Using one's own body weight as resistance allows one to develop flexibility, stamina, and strength in the context of bodyweight exercise. To get a full-body workout, nothing beats using your own body weight workouts, which may be as successful as equipment-based routines. Bodyweight exercises that train the abs, legs, chest, shoulders, & arms are abundant in the traditional 7-minute routine. Some examples are planks, squats, and push-ups.

Mastering the art of bodyweight exercise requires undivided attention to form and technique. Bodyweight exercises, when done properly, may strengthen muscles, enhance coordination, and broaden the range of motion in your joints. Bodyweight workouts are great for people of all fitness levels since they are easy to modify to increase or decrease the intensity.

2.Benefits of training without equipment

Training without equipment offers several advantages, particularly for those who want a simple, cost-effective way to stay fit. Let's look at some of the benefits of equipment-free workouts:

A.Convenience and accessibility

The ease of use is a major perk of training without tools. Going to the gym, buying pricey gym memberships or equipment like resistance bands, dumbbells, or kettlebells is unnecessary. You can exercise just about anywhere—your living area, a park, your workplace, or even a tropical island—if you have enough area to move around. Because of this, bodyweight exercises are quite convenient to include into your regular routine, and you can maintain your usual consistency no matter where you are or what time of day it is.

B.Cost-effectiveness

Fitness centre memberships and equipment may be rather pricey. Bodyweight training doesn't cost anything, which is great news for those who can't afford fancy exercise equipment. If you want to be in better shape without going into debt, it's a fantastic choice. Ideal for individuals on a short budget, it allows you to do hard and effective workouts with just your body.

C.Decreased potential for harm

There are a lot of fitness gear and devices that may help you work out, but if you don't know what you're doing, you could hurt yourself. Bodyweight workouts, on the other hand, are less likely to cause harm, provided that the exercises are executed correctly. Squats, squats and push-ups are bodyweight exercises that help you avoid overusing your joints and muscles by letting you move through their normal ranges of motion.

D.Assistive power

Strength that is useful in everyday life is known as functional strength, and it may be improved through bodyweight exercises. Natural motion patterns such as pulling, pushing, squatting, and leaping are mimicked by bodyweight motions, which include several joints and muscle groups. Strength and coordination training like this improves performance in everyday tasks like lifting, stair climbing, and athletics.

3.Essential bodyweight exercises for the S.I.T. workout

Having discussed the advantages of equipment-free training, we will now examine many essential bodyweight exercises that comprise the 7-minute S.I.T. routine. You may adjust the intensity of these workouts to suit your current fitness level, and they all work various muscle areas.

Performing squats

One of the most basic bodyweight exercises, squats work the core, glutes, hamstrings, and quadriceps. When it comes to strengthening the lower body and increasing mobility, they are among the greatest workouts. In order to squat:

1.Stand with your feet shoulder-width apart and your toes slightly pointed out.

2.Lower your body as if you were sitting back into a chair, keeping your chest upright and knees tracking over your toes.

3.Push through your heels to return to standing.

To progress, you can perform jump squats, where you explosively jump upward as you reach the standing position, or try one-legged squats (pistol squats) to increase difficulty.

B.Push-ups

One of the most well-known bodyweight exercises, push-ups target the abdominals, shoulders, and arms in addition to the core. Depending on your fitness level, you may choose from a variety of basic to difficult varieties.

1.Start in a high plank position with your hands placed slightly wider than shoulder-width apart.

2.Lower your body toward the ground by bending your elbows, keeping your body in a straight line.

3.Push through your palms to return to the starting position.

Elevated push-ups, in which you elevate your feet off the ground, and plyometric push-ups, in which you lift your wrists off the ground, are two ways to develop in this exercise. To improve form and strength, novices should try doing push-ups on knees.

C.Planks

In addition to strengthening the abdominals, the plank also works the back, legs, and shoulders. Stability and posture are greatly enhanced by it. To execute the fundamental plank:

1.Start in a forearm plank position with your elbows directly under your shoulders and your body in a straight line.

2.Hold this position while engaging your core, keeping your hips level.

3.Make sure not to let your lower back sag or your hips rise too high.

For progression, you can try side planks, which focus on the obliques, or plank variations like plank to push-up, which increase the dynamic nature of the exercise.

D.Lunges

One more great bodyweight exercise that works the glutes and legs is the lunge. They are great for enhancing coordination and balance as well. If you want to learn how to lunge:

1.Stand with your feet hip-width apart and take a large step forward with one foot.

2.Lower your body until both knees are bent at about 90 degrees.

3.Push through the heel of your front foot to return to the starting position.

To make lunges more challenging, you can add a jump between each lunge (jump lunges) or perform walking lunges, stepping forward rather than returning to the starting position after each rep.

E.Mountain climbers

Mountain climbers are great for strengthening your abs, shoulders, and legs all at once. Cardiovascular endurance is another area that they assist in. Climbers in order to make their ascent:

1.Start in a high plank position with your hands directly under your shoulders.

2.Drive one knee toward your chest, then quickly switch legs, as if you were running in place while keeping your core engaged.

3.Continue alternating legs at a fast pace.

Mountain climbers can be modified by slowing down the pace or performing them with a pause at the top of each rep to focus more on the core.

4.Structuring a 7-minute equipment-free S.I.T. workout

To create an effective 7-minute workout without equipment, you can simply adapt the exercises mentioned above to fit into the classic S.I.T. workout framework. Here's an example of how to structure an equipment-free S.I.T. workout:

- **Jumping jacks** (30 seconds)

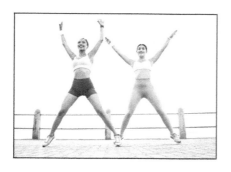

- **Push-ups** (30 seconds)

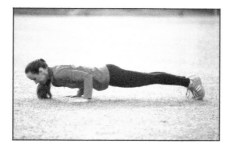

- **Squats** (30 seconds)

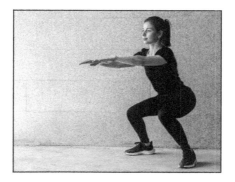

- **Plank** (30 seconds)

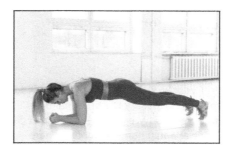

- **Lunges** (30 seconds)

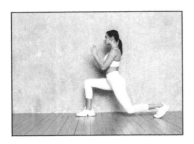

- **Mountain climbers** (30 seconds)

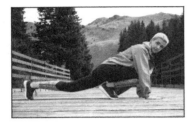

- **Burpees** (30 seconds)

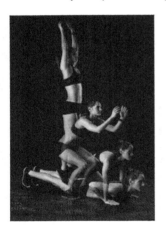

After completing each exercise, you'll have a brief rest period (usually 10 seconds) before moving to the next exercise. The goal is to keep your heart rate elevated, improving both strength and cardiovascular endurance.

5.Conclusion

You can get just as much out of your exercises even if you don't have any equipment. No gym membership or special equipment is necessary to get a total-body exercise that targets strength, stamina, and flexibility with the correct bodyweight exercises. You can always find a way to get a good exercise in without any special equipment, no matter where you are: at home, at the park, or even on vacation. Bodyweight training is a must-have for any fitness regimen due to its adaptability and accessibility; the 7-minute S.I.T. exercise is a great example of how to get a great, hard workout using only your body. You can keep becoming in shape without investing in expensive gear if you pay attention to form, intensity, and advancement.

Chapter 17: Integrating workouts into your daily routine

One of the biggest obstacles to sticking to a regular exercise program in today's hectic society is actually getting to the gym. It might be challenging to find time to exercise when you have so many other commitments, such as job, family, social events, and personal duties. Being fit, though, need not take a lot of time. Workouts, such as the 7-minute S.I.T. program, may be effortlessly included into your daily regimen with the correct frame of mind and set of techniques. To help you stay consistent and inspired on your fitness quest, this chapter will discuss practical strategies to include exercise into your daily routine.

1.Understanding the importance of consistency

Consistency is the key to achieving your fitness goals over the long run. It's more important to include exercise into your daily routine than to work out for long periods of time or to achieve perfection in each session. You may enhance your health, strength, and endurance by regularly including brief but effective exercises into your program. Because of its short length and few demands, the 7-minute S.I.T. exercise is made to be sustainable, so it's simpler for you to remain consistent.

The challenge lies in overcoming barriers such as time constraints, motivation, and competing priorities. This chapter will address these common obstacles and provide practical solutions to help you stay on track.

2.Identifying your time slots

One of the first steps to integrating workouts into your daily routine is identifying where you can realistically fit them into your day. With a short, 7-minute workout, the time commitment is minimal, so finding time shouldn't be difficult. Here are some common time slots where you can squeeze in a quick workout:

A.Early morning routine

For many people, the early morning is the best time to exercise. It's quiet, there are fewer distractions, and you can start your day with a sense of accomplishment. There are several benefits to exercising first thing in the morning, including more energy, better concentration, and a more optimistic outlook on the day ahead.

If mornings work best for you, set aside 7 minutes before breakfast to complete your S.I.T. workout. This can be as simple as rolling out of bed, putting on workout clothes, and doing your workout first thing. Since the workout is short and efficient, it won't interfere with your morning routine.

B.Lunchtime break

If mornings are too rushed or you're not a morning person, consider using your lunch break to get in a quick workout. Many workplaces offer a break between 12 and 1 p.m., and this time can be used to reset your body and mind. Instead of spending your entire break eating or lounging, dedicate just 7 minutes to a workout.

You can either do your workout in a private space at work, such as a break room or a quiet office, or you can head outside for a walk and then perform the workout outdoors if weather permits. An added bonus is that lunchtime workouts can help boost your energy for the afternoon, combatting the post-lunch slump.

C.Post-work routine

For others, the end of the workday may be the most realistic time to fit in a workout. While it's easy to get caught up in the hustle and bustle of work, making a habit of working out after your job is done can be an effective strategy. If you're someone who feels mentally drained at the end of the workday, a quick, intense 7-minute workout can actually provide a boost of energy and help clear your mind.

You can incorporate your workout into your evening routine, right after you come home and change into comfortable clothes. Whether it's before dinner or as part of your winding-down routine, it's an effective way to ensure you don't skip your workout.

D.Split sessions

Another effective strategy is splitting your workout into multiple shorter sessions throughout the day. You can perform the 7-minute S.I.T. workout twice a day, once in the morning and once in the evening, or you can break it into smaller intervals, such as 3-4 minutes of exercise after a meal or during a break at work. Splitting your sessions ensures that you stay active without feeling overwhelmed, and it can help you avoid workout fatigue.

3.Creating a habit: The power of consistency

One of the most important factors in integrating workouts into your daily routine is creating a habit. It takes time to form a consistent routine, but once it becomes a habit, it will feel like second nature. Here are some tips for turning exercise into a daily habit:

A.Set a specific time

Instead of vaguely planning to "work out sometime today," set a specific time for your 7-minute workout. Whether it's 6:00 a.m. before work or 12:30 p.m. during lunch, having a set time helps you prioritize your workout and holds you accountable. The more consistent you are with the time, the easier it becomes to stick to the routine.

B.Use reminders

It's easy to forget to work out if it's not part of your daily routine yet. Set a reminder on your phone, write it down in your calendar, or place sticky notes around your home to remind you to complete your workout. These simple prompts can be powerful tools for helping you stay on track.

C.Start small, build gradually

If you're new to exercising or have a busy lifestyle, start by committing to just a few days a week. Once you've built the habit of working out regularly, you can increase the frequency. Starting small and gradually building up to daily workouts reduces the risk of burnout and helps you stay consistent.

D.Track your progress

Another strategy to keep yourself motivated is to keep track of your progress. A visual record of your progress may be obtained by keeping a workout diary or by utilising fitness applications to record your exercises. Your likelihood of maintaining your regimen increases as you observe the cumulative effect of your regularity.

4.Overcoming common obstacles

There will inevitably be challenges along the way that make it harder to stick to your workout routine. These obstacles can include lack of motivation, time constraints, or mental fatigue. Here are some strategies to help you overcome these hurdles:

A.Lack of motivation

When motivation wanes, remember that even a short 7-minute workout is better than no workout at all. On days when motivation is low, promise yourself that you'll only do a few minutes, and once you start, you might find that you're motivated to finish the full 7 minutes. The key is to start, even when you don't feel like it.

Another effective strategy is to combine your workout with something you enjoy, such as listening to your favorite podcast, music, or an audiobook. This can make the experience more enjoyable and help distract you from any reluctance to work out.

B.Time constraints

If you feel like you're too busy to work out, remember that a 7-minute workout is one of the shortest, most time-efficient workouts you can do. To make it even easier, you can complete your workout in small, 2-3 minute chunks throughout the day. Additionally, you can use time during your commute or waiting for an appointment to squeeze in a few exercises.

C.Mental fatigue

Mental fatigue can make it difficult to find the energy to work out. However, physical activity is a great way to combat stress and improve mental clarity. If you're feeling mentally drained, a 7-minute workout can actually give you a burst of energy and help clear your mind. It might be the mental break you need to feel rejuvenated and ready to tackle the rest of your day.

5.Conclusion

Integrating workouts into your daily routine is about making exercise a non-negotiable part of your life, no matter how busy you are. With the 7-minute S.I.T. workout, you can fit in a quick, efficient workout that improves your physical health and boosts your energy. By identifying your ideal time slot, creating consistent habits, overcoming obstacles, and tracking progress, you can ensure that fitness becomes a regular part of your routine. The more you prioritize your health, the easier it will become to stay active and motivated. Ultimately, consistency is the key to success, and with just 7 minutes a day, you can achieve lasting fitness improvements.

Chapter 18: Recovery and regeneration

A lot of individuals pay close attention to how often and how hard they exercise, but often fail to provide adequate time to recuperation, which is an essential part of any effective fitness program. Maintaining your fitness level over time and avoiding injuries or burnout requires regular rest and regeneration. To make sure you're ready to take on the following workout via strength and energy, this chapter will go over the significance of wellness, how to properly rejuvenate your body after an intense activity, and how to include rest into your workout routine.

1.Why recovery matters

Muscles, joints, and the circulatory system are all put through their paces during exercise, particularly intense exercise such as the 7-minute S.I.T. routine. Microtears in muscle fibres, caused by this tension, take time to mend. Muscles strengthen and function better with time because of this mending process. If you don't give your muscles enough time to rest and recuperate after exercising, they could get injured or at least less effective.

Allowing every part of yourself to regenerate and rebuild is what recovery is all about, not simply letting your muscles repair. In order to make the most success in your fitness journey, it is essential to refill your energy stores, minimise inflammatory processes, and maintain hormonal balance.

2.Different types of recovery

Recovery can be broken down into several components, including passive recovery, active recovery, and nutritional recovery. Each of these plays a role in regenerating the body, and all are essential for balancing your training routine.

A.Passive recovery

Passive recovery refers to complete rest and relaxation, with minimal physical activity. This is often the most straightforward form of recovery, especially when your body is feeling fatigued or sore. During passive recovery, the body has time to repair the damage caused by the previous workout and adapt to the stresses placed on it.

Passive recovery can include:

- **Sleep**: Sleep is perhaps the most important recovery tool. It is during sleep that your body produces growth hormones, which are essential for muscle repair and regeneration. To give your body the time it needs to recuperate, try to get between seven and nine hours of good sleep nightly.

- If you want your muscles to be able to recover and regenerate after each workout, you need include rest days in your program. This doesn't mean you have to stay completely inactive—light walking or stretching can be beneficial—but avoid intense physical activity on rest days to give your muscles a break.

B.Active recovery

Active recuperation is doing light, low-intensity exercises to loosen up sore muscles and increase blood flow. The accumulation of lactic acid, a factor in muscular discomfort, can be mitigated by active recovery. Some things that may be done to aid in the recuperation process are:

- **Light walking or jogging**: A brisk walk or light jog helps keep your blood flowing, which can aid in the removal of waste products and provide nutrients to muscles for repair.
- **Cycling**: Low-intensity cycling is another excellent active recovery exercise, as it engages your lower body muscles and increases circulation without putting too much strain on them.
- **Yoga or stretching**: To relax, loosen up, and become more flexible, try some light yoga or stretching. Participating in these pursuits can boost health and happiness in general.

C.Nutritional recovery

A healthy diet is an important part of getting better. For optimal energy restoration, muscle regeneration, and post-workout recovery, your body need a certain set of nutrients. Making sure your body gets the nutrients it needs after exercise is crucial, and not only in the moments after a workout.

Key aspects of nutritional recovery include:

- **Protein**: Building and repairing muscles need protein. Consuming a meal high in protein or snack after exercise is essential for repairing muscle fibres that were damaged during the session. The goal is to consume 20-30 grammes for protein between 30-60 minutes after your workout is over.

- Carbohydrates: The body's main energy store, glycogen, may be restocked by carbohydrates. To replenish energy and be ready for the next session, eat a reasonable amount of nutritious carbs after your workout.

- Healthy fats, such as those in almonds, avocados, and olive oil, play a key role in hormone balance, joint repair, and general well-being. Incorporating them into your post-workout meals will provide the best possible recuperation.

- Staying hydrated is crucial for a speedy recovery, yet it often gets neglected. Sweat is a major fluid loss during exercise, therefore it's important to drink enough of water to stay hydrated and aid in recovery. Always stay hydrated, whether it's before, during, or after your workout. Depending on the severity of your perspiration, it may be necessary to replenish your electrolytes as well.

3.Importance of stretching and mobility

Stretching, despite its apparent simplicity, is an essential part of the healing and regenerative processes. Muscles may be lengthened, flexibility increased, and injury risk decreased by stretching. When you work out, your muscles tend to be tight, but stretching may help loosen them up and keep them from being stiff again.

A. Static elongation

To improve flexibility and reduce muscular tension, static stretching is doing a stretch while holding it for a certain amount of time, often 15 to 30 seconds. When you want to make sure the muscles are comfortable and supple after a workout, static stretches are a must.

Some beneficial static stretches include:

- **Hamstring stretch**: Stretching the hamstrings can help alleviate tightness in the legs after exercises like squats or lunges.
- **Hip flexor stretch**: Tight hip flexors can develop from squatting or sitting for long periods, so stretching the hip flexors can promote better posture and mobility.

- **Quadriceps stretch**: Stretching the quads is particularly important after leg-intensive exercises to reduce tightness and promote knee health.

B.Dynamic stretching and mobility exercises

Before an exercise, it's common practice to do dynamic stretching to improve flexibility, range of motion, and blood circulation. When it comes to protecting your joints and increasing their range of motion, mobility exercises are your best bet.

Common dynamic stretches and mobility exercises include:

- **Leg swings**: A great way to warm up the hips and legs before a workout.
- **Arm circles**: These activate the shoulders and upper body.
- **Hip circles**: Excellent for warming up the hip joints and promoting flexibility.

4.The role of mindfulness and stress reduction

Mental healing is an integral part of the healing process, just as much as physical regeneration. Mental and physical stress can raise cortisol levels and promote inflammation, which can slow down the healing process. Reducing stress and improving overall healing can be achieved via the incorporation of mindfulness and relaxation practices.

A.Meditation

Meditation is a powerful tool for reducing mental stress and promoting relaxation. Even just 5-10 minutes of meditation per day can lower cortisol levels, improve sleep quality, and enhance overall mental well-being. Meditation also has the added benefit of helping you remain focused and mindful during your workouts.

B.Breathing exercises

Breathing exercises are another effective way to reduce stress and promote relaxation. Deep belly breathing or box breathing techniques can activate the parasympathetic nervous system, which is responsible for rest and recovery. Practicing deep breathing for a few minutes after your workout can speed up the regeneration process and help your body relax.

5.Listening to your body

Being attuned to your body's signals is the single most critical component of a successful recovery. Pay attention to your body and put rest first if you're feeling mentally or physically exhausted. Your emotional and physical well-being might take a hit if you overtrain and don't give yourself enough time to recover.

Staying injury-free and achieving steady development requires paying close attention to your body's signals and prioritising rehabilitation.

6.Conclusion

The time spent resting and regenerating between exercises is crucial. Fatigue, injuries, and decreased performance might result from an inadequate recuperation period. You may improve your fitness results in the long run and speed up the healing process by exercising regularly, eating well, staying hydrated, stretching, and practicing mindfulness.

You should incorporate recuperation into your entire fitness regimen since it is an method, not a one-and-done deal. Always be prepared for the following workout by making recuperation a top priority and listening to your body's demands.

Chapter 19: Staying motivated long-term

People frequently attribute their level of achievement in the fitness industry to their level of motivation. It's the driving force behind your exercises, whether you're feeling like taking a break or not. For the most part, though, maintaining motivation over the long haul is a major obstacle. Inspiration can come and go, and the thrill of beginning a new exercise program can quickly wear off, leaving you to wonder what's holding you back.

Whether you're doing a 7-minute S.I.T. exercise or something else entirely, this chapter will cover some practical tactics to help you stay motivated and devoted to your fitness objectives. A mix of mental adjustments, methods for establishing attainable goals, systems for holding yourself accountable, and approaches to making exercise fun and sustainable can keep you motivated over the long haul. Now, let's explore some ways to maintain that drive.

.

1.Setting clear and achievable goals

Having well-defined, attainable objectives is a great motivator in the long run. It is much simpler to maintain concentration and drive when you know exactly what you want to accomplish. Make sure your exercise goals are reasonable and measurable by setting them with the SMART framework: specific, measurable, realisable, and Time-bound.

A.Short-term vs. long-term goals

While long-term goals are important for giving you an overall direction, short-term goals help you stay motivated by providing immediate milestones to achieve. For example, a long-term goal could be to improve your cardiovascular fitness over six months, while a short-term goal might be to complete the 7-minute S.I.T. workout three times a week for a month.

Short-term goals create a sense of accomplishment, making the long-term goal feel more attainable. Each time you achieve a short-term goal, it reinforces your commitment to your fitness routine and helps maintain motivation.

B.Track your progress

Tracking progress not only keeps you motivated but also allows you to reflect on how far you've come. Whether you use a fitness app, a workout journal, or simply jot down notes about each session, keeping track of your workouts, times, or performance helps you see improvement over time. Progress might look like completing an additional round of exercises or feeling less fatigued during the 7-minute workout. These small wins are important reminders of how your dedication is paying off.

2.Find your "Why"

Motivation often fades when you lose sight of the deeper reasons why you started working out in the first place. To stay motivated long-term, it's essential to identify your personal "why"—the emotional and psychological reasons behind your fitness goals. This could be anything from wanting to feel more confident, to improving your health, or simply having more energy to play with your kids.

By understanding and reconnecting with your "why," you create a solid foundation that can keep you going even when motivation wanes. Write your "why" down and place it somewhere visible to remind yourself of the bigger picture. Whenever you feel discouraged, revisiting your reasons for starting can reignite your passion and help you stay on track.

3.Make workouts enjoyable

One of the biggest challenges to staying motivated long-term is the potential monotony of a fitness routine. If you don't enjoy your workouts, you're less likely to stick with them. That's why it's important to make your 7-minute S.I.T. workouts—or any fitness regimen—fun and engaging.

A.Vary your routine

Even though the 7-minute S.I.T. workout is efficient, incorporating variations can keep things fresh and exciting. You can modify the exercises, add new movements, or change the order of exercises. You can also introduce new forms of exercise into your week, such as yoga, strength training, or cycling, to keep your routine diverse and interesting.

Variety also prevents boredom and helps you avoid hitting a plateau, which can happen when you do the same routine repeatedly without any changes. By mixing up your workouts, you'll challenge your body in different ways, which can lead to faster progress and more long-term motivation.

B.Listen to music or podcasts

Sometimes the simplest changes can make your workout more enjoyable. Listening to your favorite playlist, podcast, or audiobook can keep you entertained and distracted during the 7-minute workout. Music with an upbeat tempo, for instance, can energize you and keep you moving at a steady pace. Podcasts or audiobooks provide the opportunity to learn something new or immerse yourself in a story while getting fit.

C.Reward yourself

Another way to make your workouts enjoyable is by giving yourself a reward for completing them. This could be a post-workout treat, a relaxing bath, or a night out with friends. By pairing your workout with something you enjoy, you'll associate exercise with positive emotions, making it more likely that you'll keep coming back for more.

4.Create a support system

One of the most powerful motivators is having a strong support system. Whether it's a workout buddy, a fitness community, or an online group, being part of a group that encourages and holds you accountable can make a huge difference in your ability to stay motivated.

A.Workout partners

Exercising with a friend or family member can make workouts more enjoyable and social. You can cheer each other on, challenge one another, and celebrate progress together. When you have someone relying on you to show up, you're more likely to stay consistent with your routine.

B.Online communities

If you don't have a workout partner nearby, consider joining an online fitness community. Many fitness apps, social media groups, or forums provide spaces where you can share your progress, ask questions, and gain motivation from others. Being part of a supportive online community can help you stay accountable and provide you with valuable tips to improve your workouts.

C.Accountability partners

Having someone hold you accountable for your fitness routine can make a huge difference. This could be a coach, a friend, or even a family member who checks in with you regularly to see if you're sticking to your goals. Knowing that someone is watching your progress or expecting you to report back can provide extra motivation to stay committed.

5.Be kind to yourself

Staying motivated doesn't mean being perfect. Life will throw challenges your way, and sometimes you might miss a workout, feel too tired to exercise, or fall short of your goals. It's important to be kind to yourself during these moments. Instead of beating yourself up over missed workouts, view setbacks as opportunities to learn and improve. Remember that one missed session doesn't define your overall progress, and you can always get back on track.

A.Practice self-compassion

Self-compassion is about treating yourself with the same kindness and understanding that you would extend to a friend. When things don't go as planned, instead of criticizing yourself, offer encouragement. Recognize that setbacks are a normal part of any fitness journey and that success is about long-term consistency, not perfection.

B.Celebrate small wins

Every small accomplishment is a step toward your ultimate goal. Whether it's increasing the intensity of your workout, finishing your first 7-minute session without stopping, or simply sticking to your routine for a week, celebrate these milestones. Each time you achieve something, take a moment to appreciate your effort and progress. Recognizing these victories will help you maintain a positive mindset and reinforce your motivation to continue.

6.Finding balance

While it's important to stay motivated, it's equally important to avoid burnout. Overtraining, constant pressure to perform, and lack of rest can lead to physical and mental exhaustion. To stay motivated over the long term, find a balance between pushing yourself and allowing for recovery. Take rest days when needed, listen to your body, and be patient with your progress.

Balancing your workouts with recovery and other aspects of your life will keep you refreshed, focused, and motivated in the long run. If you're constantly pushing yourself to the limit without proper rest, you risk losing motivation and burning out.

7.Conclusion

Staying motivated long-term is a challenge, but it's one that can be overcome with the right strategies and mindset. By setting clear goals, finding your "why," making workouts enjoyable, creating a support system, being kind to yourself, and balancing your efforts with adequate rest, you can maintain your motivation and stay committed to your fitness routine. Remember, fitness is a marathon, not a sprint, and long-term success comes from consistency, patience, and a positive mindset. Stay focused, celebrate your progress, and keep pushing forward toward your goals. With time and dedication, the results will follow, and you'll build a fitness routine that you can sustain for years to come.

Chapter 20: S.I.T. for specific goals

One of the greatest advantages of the S.I.T. (Short Intensity Training) workout is its adaptability. While the workout is structured to be effective for general fitness, it can also be tailored to target specific goals. Whether your focus is weight loss, muscle building, improving cardiovascular health, or boosting athletic performance, S.I.T. can be modified to fit your unique objectives. In this chapter, we will explore how to adjust the S.I.T. workout to align with various fitness goals, ensuring that you make the most of your short, yet effective workout sessions.

1.S.I.T. for weight loss

For many, the primary reason for starting a fitness routine is to lose weight. The challenge often lies in finding an exercise routine that fits into a busy schedule and remains sustainable over the long term. The 7-minute S.I.T. workout is an ideal choice for those looking to shed pounds, as it combines high-intensity exercises with minimal time commitment.

A.The role of high-intensity interval training (HIIT)

The 7-minute S.I.T. workout is a form of high-intensity interval training (HIIT). HIIT has been proven to be highly effective for fat loss due to its ability to increase the body's calorie burn both during and after exercise. This is known as the afterburn effect or excess post-exercise oxygen consumption (EPOC), which helps the body continue to burn calories at a higher rate even after the workout is over.

When designed for weight loss, S.I.T. should incorporate exercises that elevate the heart rate and maximize calorie expenditure. Exercises like jumping jacks, mountain climbers, burpees, and high knees are great examples of movements that can be used to push your body into the fat-burning zone.

B.Increasing intensity

For weight loss, it's essential to push the body beyond its normal capacity during each 7-minute session. This can be achieved by increasing the intensity of the exercises. You can do this by:

- **Performing exercises at a faster pace**: For example, instead of performing bodyweight squats at a moderate pace, do them explosively to increase heart rate and calorie burn.
- **Incorporating plyometric movements**: Plyometric exercises, such as jump squats, tuck jumps, and box jumps, are effective in burning fat while also increasing strength and endurance.
- **Shortening rest periods**: The less rest you take between exercises, the more intense the workout becomes. Try limiting rest periods to 5-10 seconds or, in some cases, eliminating them entirely for an even more challenging session.

C.Combining with nutrition

While S.I.T. is highly effective for weight loss, nutrition plays an equally important role. To optimize fat loss, ensure that you are eating a well-balanced diet with a slight caloric deficit. Focus on whole foods such as lean proteins, fruits, vegetables, and complex carbohydrates, while minimizing processed foods, refined sugars, and excessive fats. A healthy diet combined with your S.I.T. workouts will help you achieve the best results.

2.S.I.T. for muscle building

Building muscle requires a slightly different approach to S.I.T. than weight loss. While S.I.T. can certainly help with muscle endurance and toning, those looking to build muscle mass will need to focus on strength and resistance training. Fortunately, S.I.T. can be modified to help build lean muscle, especially if paired with the right exercises and a well-rounded workout routine.

A. Incorporating strength training

To target muscle growth through S.I.T., you should incorporate exercises that engage large muscle groups and utilize bodyweight resistance. This might include:

- **Push-ups**: A classic bodyweight exercise that works the chest, shoulders, and triceps.
- **Squats and lunges**: Lower-body exercises that engage the quadriceps, hamstrings, and glutes.
- **Planks**: Core-strengthening exercises that also engage the shoulders and glutes.
- **Dips**: Target the triceps, chest, and shoulders.

While these exercises can help to build muscle through bodyweight resistance, for greater muscle development, you can also incorporate additional equipment such as dumbbells, resistance bands, or kettlebells. Using weights will create more resistance and allow for progressive overload, a principle essential for muscle growth.

B. Progressive overload

Progressive overload refers to gradually increasing the intensity of your workouts to continue making progress. This is key to building muscle and strength. In the context of S.I.T., progressive overload can be achieved by:

- **Increasing the number of sets and reps**: Over time, gradually add more rounds to your workout or increase the repetitions of each exercise.
- **Adding weights**: Incorporating dumbbells or kettlebells into exercises like squats, lunges, and push-ups will increase the resistance and stimulate muscle growth.
- **Reducing rest time**: By shortening rest periods between sets, you can increase the intensity of your workouts, which will encourage more muscle development.

C. Adequate recovery

When working on building muscle, rest and recovery are just as important as the workout itself. Make sure to give your muscles time to repair and grow. Adequate sleep, a balanced diet rich in protein, and rest days between intense S.I.T. sessions are essential for muscle development.

---

3. S.I.T. for cardiovascular health

S.I.T. is excellent for improving cardiovascular health due to its high intensity and the way it challenges the heart and lungs. The rapid bursts of effort followed by short periods of rest provide the cardiovascular system with an excellent workout that improves heart health, lung capacity, and overall endurance.

A. The benefits of interval training

S.I.T. mimics the benefits of traditional cardio exercises, such as running or cycling, but in a shorter time frame. The intense intervals increase the heart rate, stimulating the cardiovascular system and improving heart function. Research shows that interval training can improve VO2 max (the amount of oxygen your body can utilize during exercise), which is a key indicator of cardiovascular fitness.

To tailor your S.I.T. workouts for cardiovascular health, focus on exercises that keep your heart rate elevated for the duration of the workout. Some of the best exercises for cardiovascular conditioning include:

- **Jumping jacks**

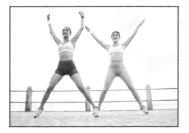

- **Burpees**

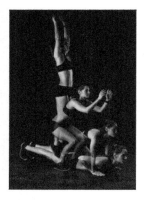

- **High knees**

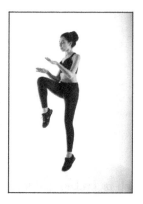

- **Mountain climbers**

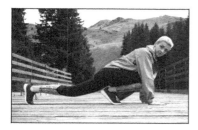

- **Skater hops**

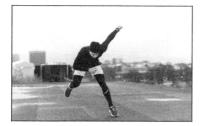

These exercises elevate your heart rate and improve cardiovascular endurance, helping you build a healthier heart over time.

B.Frequency and consistency

For optimal cardiovascular health, aim to perform S.I.T. workouts at least 3-5 times per week. Consistency is key to reaping the benefits of improved cardiovascular health. Additionally, incorporate variety into your routine to keep things fresh and challenge your heart in different ways. By varying the exercises and increasing the intensity, you ensure that your cardiovascular system continues to adapt and improve.

4.S.I.T. for athletic performance

Athletes looking to improve their performance can benefit greatly from S.I.T., as it is designed to improve both strength and endurance. The intensity of S.I.T. workouts mimics the physical demands of many sports, where short bursts of effort are followed by periods of rest or lower intensity. By increasing power, agility, and stamina, S.I.T. can help athletes become better at their sport.

A.Plyometric and explosive training

To enhance athletic performance, incorporate explosive movements such as jump squats, sprints, and box jumps into your S.I.T. routine. These exercises improve explosive power, which is essential for sports like basketball, soccer, football, and track and field. They engage fast-twitch muscle fibers, which are responsible for rapid movements and bursts of speed.

B.Agility and speed

S.I.T. can also help improve agility and speed through quick direction changes and high-speed movements. Exercises like ladder drills, cone drills, and shuttle runs are excellent for improving your ability to quickly accelerate, decelerate, and change direction—skills that are crucial for sports performance.

C.Conditioning for sport-specific movements

Finally, for sport-specific performance, it's important to tailor your S.I.T. workout to mimic the movements involved in your sport. For example, football players may focus on exercises that build lower body strength and explosiveness, while swimmers may target upper body and core exercises. S.I.T. workouts can be easily adjusted to align with the unique demands of your sport.

5.Conclusion

The 7-minute S.I.T. workout is not only a time-efficient exercise routine, but it can also be adapted to suit a wide range of specific fitness goals. Whether you are looking to lose weight, build muscle, improve cardiovascular health, or enhance athletic performance, S.I.T. can be tailored to meet your needs. By modifying the intensity, focusing on different exercises, and maintaining a consistent routine, you can achieve significant progress toward any fitness goal.

Ultimately, the beauty of S.I.T. lies in its versatility. It's a customizable approach to fitness that can evolve as your goals shift, allowing you to maintain motivation and continue to see results over the long term.

Chapter 21: Training in small spaces

In a world where space often comes at a premium, particularly in urban environments, finding the room to exercise can sometimes feel like a challenge. Whether you live in a small apartment, have a crowded office, or simply lack a dedicated home gym, limited space doesn't have to be a barrier to achieving your fitness goals. Training in small spaces is entirely possible, and the 7-minute S.I.T. workout is particularly well-suited to this type of environment.

In this chapter, we will explore how to maximize your small space for effective workouts, provide creative solutions to limited room, and demonstrate that you can achieve your fitness goals regardless of the size of your surroundings.

1.The benefits of small space training

Before diving into specific strategies for making the most of your limited space, it's important to understand the benefits of training in small spaces:

A.Convenience

One of the biggest advantages of training in small spaces is convenience. Whether it's your living room, bedroom, or even a small corner of your office, small space workouts make it easy to fit exercise into your day. There are no long commutes to the gym, no need to wait for equipment, and no distractions. You can work out whenever you want, for as long as you need, and it's just a matter of getting started. With a minimal setup, small space workouts can be done quickly and efficiently, making them a great option for busy individuals.

B.Flexibility

When working out in a small space, you're not limited to specific hours of operation, like a gym might be. The flexibility of being able to exercise whenever and wherever you choose means you can fit workouts into any part of your day. Additionally, small space workouts can be performed in various locations, whether at home, in a hotel room while traveling, or in a small apartment—allowing for consistency regardless of your location.

C.Less distraction

Unlike a gym where the environment can be overwhelming, a small space can provide a more focused, quieter setting for exercise. Without the distractions of other people, loud music, or waiting for machines, you can concentrate entirely on your workout. This focused environment can lead to better results, as you're less likely to be interrupted or sidetracked.

2.Designing your S.I.T. workout in small spaces

The key to successfully training in a small space is knowing how to make the most of the area you have. With the right mindset, you'll see that you don't need a lot of room to get an effective workout. The 7-minute S.I.T. workout is particularly adaptable to small spaces, as the exercises require minimal equipment and can often be done in a small footprint.

A.Bodyweight exercises

The 7-minute S.I.T. workout is primarily made up of bodyweight exercises, which are ideal for small spaces. These exercises do not require much room and can be done with just your body as the resistance. Some examples of bodyweight exercises that can be performed in a limited space include:

- **Jumping jacks**: A simple full-body exercise that can be performed in any room.

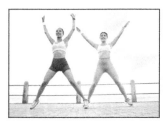

- **Mountain climbers**: A core exercise that only requires enough space to extend your legs in a plank position.

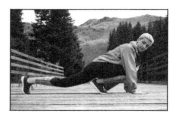

- **Push-ups**: A fundamental bodyweight exercise that can be done on the floor.

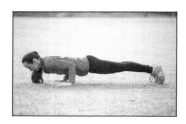

- **Squats**: Lower body exercise requiring no equipment and little space.

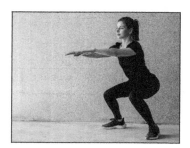

- **Planks**: A core-stabilizing move that requires only a small area on the floor.

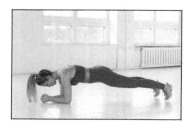

- **Burpees**: Full-body exercise with jumping motions that can be done in confined spaces.

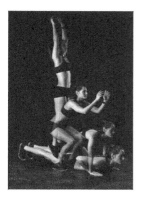

When performing these exercises, make sure that the area you are working in is clear of obstructions to avoid injury. For exercises that require jumping, like jump squats or burpees, take care to jump softly and avoid hitting walls or furniture.

B.Use minimal equipment

While the 7-minute S.I.T. workout doesn't require much equipment, if you're looking to increase the intensity or target specific muscle groups, you can incorporate some basic gear. Opt for items that are easy to store and won't take up much space. Some great options include:

- **Resistance bands**: These are compact and versatile tools that can be used to add resistance to bodyweight exercises, such as squats, lunges, and chest presses.
- **Dumbbells**: If you have space for a pair of light dumbbells, you can incorporate them into your workout to increase strength-building efforts. Dumbbells are small and easy to store.
- **Kettlebells**: A single kettlebell can be used for exercises like kettlebell swings, goblet squats, and more, while taking up very little room.
- **Yoga mats**: If you're doing floor-based exercises like planks, push-ups, or stretching, a mat provides cushioning and ensures comfort during your workout.

All of these items can be used within a small workout area and can be easily stored when not in use, allowing for more space when necessary.

C.Focus on vertical and horizontal movements

To optimize your limited space, focus on exercises that emphasize both vertical and horizontal movements. This will help you maximize the area you're using without requiring too much floor space. Here are some ideas:

- **Vertical movements**: Exercises that involve moving upward or involving jumping can be done in a confined space. Jumping jacks, squat jumps, and high knees work great in small spaces.
- **Horizontal movements**: Movements that require you to lie down, such as push-ups, planks, and leg raises, are perfect for floor-based exercises in a limited area.

3.Adapting the 7-minute S.I.T. workout for small spaces

The beauty of the S.I.T. workout lies in its adaptability. With just 7 minutes of exercise, you can get an intense and effective workout regardless of the space you have. Here's how you can adapt the workout for even the smallest spaces:

A.Modifying movements

If you find that a particular exercise is difficult to perform due to space constraints, you can modify it. For example, if you're doing burpees but have limited room to jump, you can eliminate the jump and simply perform a squat thrust (also known as a half burpee) instead. Similarly, if you're doing mountain climbers but need a smaller range of motion, simply adjust the movement by bringing your knees up only slightly.

B.Performing circuit training

If you're limited in space, one of the best ways to get the most out of your workout is by performing circuit training. Circuit training is where you cycle through multiple exercises with minimal rest in between, keeping your heart rate elevated while targeting different muscle groups. This works well with the 7-minute S.I.T. workout as it uses bodyweight exercises that flow seamlessly from one to another. You can modify the order of exercises or include a few additional movements to challenge your body and prevent monotony.

4.Creating a workout schedule for small spaces

The key to any successful fitness regimen is consistency. Training in small spaces can be incredibly convenient, but it's important to establish a regular workout schedule to ensure you stay on track. Here's how you can make training in small spaces a regular part of your life:

A.Set a routine

Create a set schedule for when you'll complete your S.I.T. workouts. Whether it's first thing in the morning, during your lunch break, or after work, setting aside time to exercise every day will help make it a habit. With just 7 minutes, it's easy to fit in a quick workout, and you'll be more motivated knowing you don't need to carve out a lot of time for it.

B.Use a timer or app

Since S.I.T. workouts are timed, using a timer or a fitness app can help you stay on track. Many fitness apps are designed specifically for short, high-intensity workouts and will guide you through each exercise with pre-set timers, allowing you to focus entirely on your workout. This is particularly helpful when working out in small spaces, as you can be more efficient with your time.

5.Conclusion

Training in small spaces is not only feasible but also effective. The 7-minute S.I.T. workout is perfectly suited to small environments because it doesn't require a lot of room or equipment. With the right mindset and a few clever modifications, you can create a full-body workout routine that maximizes every square inch of your space. By focusing on bodyweight exercises, minimal equipment, and using your space creatively, you can achieve your fitness goals no matter how small your workout area may be. Whether you're training in your apartment, at a hotel, or even in a corner of your office, there's always time and space for fitness with S.I.T.

Chapter 22: S.I.T. for all ages

One of the most attractive features of the 7-minute S.I.T. workout is its adaptability. It's not just a workout for young adults or athletes—S.I.T. can be tailored to meet the needs of people of all ages. Whether you're a child, a senior citizen, or somewhere in between, the principles behind S.I.T. (Short Intensity Training) can be applied to improve fitness at any stage of life. In this chapter, we will explore how S.I.T. workouts can be beneficial for different age groups and how you can adjust your routine based on your unique needs and abilities.

1.S.I.T. for children and adolescents

Exercise is essential for the development of children and adolescents, promoting healthy growth, building strength, and enhancing motor skills. The 7-minute S.I.T. workout can provide a quick and enjoyable way for younger individuals to stay active without requiring a significant time commitment.

A.Promoting healthy growth

For children and adolescents, physical activity is crucial for building strong bones, muscles, and joints. Engaging in regular exercise helps children maintain a healthy weight, improve posture, and develop fine motor skills. S.I.T. workouts can help children achieve all of these benefits while also keeping them engaged with fun and varied movements.

S.I.T. exercises like jumping jacks, mountain climbers, high knees, and bodyweight squats can improve coordination, balance, and strength. These activities mimic the natural movements children engage in during play and sports, making them both fun and beneficial for their development.

B.Energy expenditure and weight management

As children and adolescents grow, managing their energy balance is important for preventing obesity and promoting healthy weight management. S.I.T. workouts offer an excellent way to burn calories and boost metabolism, contributing to healthy weight control. Short bursts of high-intensity exercise help regulate energy expenditure and foster a positive relationship with physical activity from a young age.

Because S.I.T. workouts are quick, children are more likely to stick with them. These short, structured routines can be done in the comfort of the home or even in a small outdoor area. Using exercise as a fun family activity can help instill lifelong habits that support good health.

C.Mental and emotional well-being

Exercise is not just good for the body; it's also beneficial for mental health. For children and adolescents, physical activity can reduce stress, improve sleep, and increase self-esteem. Studies have shown that regular exercise, such as S.I.T., can improve focus and academic performance by boosting the brain's ability to function and concentrate. The fun and challenging nature of S.I.T. workouts helps children develop a positive attitude toward fitness and well-being.

2.S.I.T. for young adults

For young adults, S.I.T. workouts can be an effective way to maintain or improve fitness levels, especially for those with busy schedules. In their 20s and 30s, individuals often juggle work, social commitments, and personal life, making it difficult to find the time to work out. The time-efficient nature of the 7-minute S.I.T. workout allows young adults to fit exercise into their day without disrupting their routines.

A.Enhancing cardiovascular health

Young adults are in a prime position to build cardiovascular fitness, and incorporating S.I.T. into their routine can be a powerful tool for improving heart health. High-intensity interval training (HIIT), which is the foundation of the S.I.T. workout, increases heart rate and improves VO2 max (a measure of cardiovascular fitness). Regular S.I.T. sessions help reduce the risk of heart disease, improve blood circulation, and maintain healthy blood pressure levels.

S.I.T. exercises like burpees, jumping jacks, and high knees raise the heart rate quickly, stimulating the cardiovascular system and enhancing endurance. As a result, young adults can stay fit, healthy, and energetic while developing lifelong cardiovascular resilience.

B.Building strength and muscle tone

In addition to cardiovascular health, S.I.T. workouts are highly effective for building muscle strength and tone. Bodyweight exercises such as squats, lunges, push-ups, and planks target multiple muscle groups, helping young adults increase lean muscle mass. For those looking to improve overall strength and definition, adding resistance through dumbbells, kettlebells, or resistance bands can further challenge the muscles and stimulate muscle growth.

Since S.I.T. workouts focus on large muscle groups and engage the core, young adults will benefit from improved muscle endurance, strength, and mobility. These benefits translate to better athletic performance and a more active lifestyle.

C.Mental clarity and stress relief

The demands of young adulthood, including work, relationships, and personal responsibilities, can sometimes lead to high levels of stress. Regular exercise, including S.I.T., is an effective way to relieve tension and boost mental well-being. Physical activity triggers the release of endorphins, which are natural mood lifters, reducing feelings of anxiety and depression.

Incorporating S.I.T. into a daily routine can serve as a mental reset, providing a much-needed break from the pressures of life. With just seven minutes of effort, young adults can experience an improved mood, enhanced mental clarity, and a greater sense of accomplishment.

3.S.I.T. for middle-aged adults

As people enter their 40s and 50s, their bodies begin to experience the effects of aging, such as muscle loss, a slowing metabolism, and reduced flexibility. S.I.T. workouts can be an excellent tool to combat these changes and maintain a high level of fitness, strength, and health.

A.Preventing muscle loss and osteoporosis

One of the major concerns as individuals age is the loss of muscle mass and bone density. S.I.T. workouts that incorporate strength training exercises, such as squats, lunges, and push-ups, help to counteract muscle loss and promote lean muscle development. Regular weight-bearing exercise also helps maintain bone density, reducing the risk of osteoporosis.

Incorporating resistance bands or weights into your S.I.T. workouts is a great way to ensure that your muscles are continuously challenged, leading to muscle growth and better bone health. This can also help with maintaining functional strength, making it easier to perform daily tasks and reduce the risk of falls.

B.Boosting metabolism

Metabolism naturally slows down with age, which can contribute to weight gain and difficulty losing fat. The high-intensity nature of S.I.T. helps to increase metabolic rate both during and after the workout. This "afterburn" effect, or excess post-exercise oxygen consumption (EPOC), ensures that your body continues to burn calories at a higher rate even after you've finished your workout.

S.I.T. is especially beneficial for middle-aged adults who are trying to maintain or lose weight. Short, intense bursts of exercise rev up the metabolism and promote fat loss, without the need for hours of cardio. With only 7 minutes of exercise, the time commitment is minimal, making it an ideal choice for busy schedules.

C.Enhancing mental agility

In addition to physical benefits, exercise also improves cognitive function. For middle-aged adults, staying mentally sharp is just as important as physical health. Regular exercise, such as S.I.T., increases blood flow to the brain, which supports memory, focus, and mental clarity. Research shows that people who engage in regular physical activity are at a lower risk of developing cognitive decline and conditions such as dementia.

Short, intense workouts like S.I.T. provide mental stimulation while also giving you the emotional benefits of stress reduction and increased confidence.

4.S.I.T. for seniors

For older adults, staying active is crucial to maintaining independence, mobility, and overall health. While high-intensity training may sound intimidating, the beauty of the 7-minute S.I.T. workout is that it can be adjusted to suit people of all fitness levels, including seniors. With proper modifications and focus on mobility and functional movements, S.I.T. can improve strength, balance, and quality of life for older adults.

A.Improving mobility and flexibility

As people age, joint stiffness and limited range of motion can make movement more difficult. S.I.T. workouts can improve mobility by incorporating gentle yet effective exercises like seated leg raises, chair squats, and standing marches. These low-impact exercises improve joint health, increase flexibility, and help older adults stay mobile and agile.

Gentle stretching exercises, when included as part of a S.I.T. routine, also promote flexibility and reduce the risk of falls by improving balance and coordination.

B.Enhancing balance and coordination

Falls are a major concern for older adults, and improving balance and coordination is one of the best ways to reduce the risk. S.I.T. workouts that include balance-focused exercises like single-leg stands, side leg raises, and step-ups help seniors maintain strength and stability, improving their ability to move confidently throughout the day.

Strengthening exercises such as squats and lunges also improve lower-body strength, contributing to better balance and stability.

C.Supporting heart health

Cardiovascular health remains a key concern as individuals age. The heart tends to become less efficient with age, and seniors may be at greater risk of heart disease, high blood pressure, and stroke. Regular S.I.T. workouts, even at a moderate intensity, can help improve heart health. Cardiovascular exercises like high knees, walking lunges, or light jogging are all excellent for increasing heart rate and boosting circulation.

Incorporating just a few minutes of S.I.T. into a daily routine can lower the risk of heart disease and promote healthier blood pressure levels.

5.Conclusion

S.I.T. workouts are suitable for individuals of all ages, from children to seniors. The key to success lies in modifying the exercises to meet the needs and abilities of each age group. Whether you're aiming to improve strength, cardiovascular health, mobility, or mental well-being, S.I.T. provides a flexible and effective approach to fitness. By adapting the workout to your specific age-related needs, you can stay active, healthy, and strong throughout your life.

Chapter 23: Mental focus and mindfulness in training

Training your body is only one piece of the puzzle when it comes to fitness. The power of mental focus and mindfulness plays an equally important role in the success of any workout regimen. When you incorporate mental discipline into your training, you not only maximize your physical potential, but you also create a deeper connection between your mind and body. The 7-minute S.I.T. workout, with its emphasis on intensity, short intervals, and efficient movement, is an ideal platform for building mental focus and practicing mindfulness. In this chapter, we will explore how mental focus and mindfulness can elevate your workout experience, and how these concepts can be integrated into your daily fitness routine.

1.The role of mental focus in fitness

Mental focus is the ability to concentrate your attention on the task at hand without being distracted by external stimuli or wandering thoughts. In the context of a workout, it means giving your full attention to each movement, your body's sensations, and the progression of your exercises. Mental focus can significantly enhance the quality of your workout, improving both performance and outcomes.

A.Staying present during workouts

One of the most significant aspects of mental focus is learning to stay present. In today's fast-paced world, distractions are everywhere, from smartphones to to-do lists. However, being mentally present during a workout allows you to get the most out of each movement. In a S.I.T. workout, where you perform high-intensity exercises with short rest intervals, focusing your mind on the task at hand is crucial. When you are fully engaged, you're more likely to push through the discomfort of intense movements and get the most benefit from your workout.

For example, during jumping jacks, focus on the rhythm of your movements, how your body feels, and the sensation of your feet lifting off the ground. Pay attention to your breathing, the tightening of your core, and the engagement of your muscles. The more present you are, the better the results.

B.Improved performance

Focusing your attention on each exercise also enhances your performance. When you're mindful of your technique, you're more likely to perform exercises with proper form, which reduces the risk of injury and increases the effectiveness of the workout. Whether it's a squat, a push-up, or a mountain climber, attention to form and alignment can ensure you're targeting the right muscles and moving in a way that maximizes the benefits.

By concentrating on the muscle groups you're working, you enhance the mind-muscle connection, which is key to improving strength, endurance, and overall performance. When you zone out or lose focus, it can lead to sloppy technique, reduced intensity, and missed opportunities for muscle activation.

C.Overcoming mental barriers

In high-intensity workouts like S.I.T., mental barriers can be one of the biggest challenges. You may find yourself wanting to quit during the most intense moments, but by training your mental focus, you can push past those limits. Developing the mental strength to overcome discomfort and fatigue is crucial for achieving better results and progressing in your fitness journey.

By cultivating a focused mindset, you can learn to ignore the voice in your head telling you to stop and instead focus on the next repetition, the next breath, and the next goal. The mental discipline you develop during a S.I.T. workout can transfer to other areas of your life, helping you tackle challenges with a positive and determined attitude.

2.Mindfulness: Bringing awareness to your workout

Mindfulness is the practice of paying full attention to the present moment without judgment. While it is often associated with meditation, mindfulness can also be applied to physical activities, including exercise. When you approach your workout with a mindful attitude, you become more aware of your body's movements, your breath, and the sensations that arise throughout the workout. Mindfulness allows you to engage in your workout more deeply, creating a holistic experience that is both physically and mentally rewarding.

A.Awareness of breath

One of the easiest ways to introduce mindfulness into your S.I.T. workout is by focusing on your breath. Breathing is a natural rhythm that ties the mind and body together. When we focus on our breath, we enhance our sense of calm, reduce stress, and improve our exercise performance. Proper breathing during high-intensity intervals helps regulate your heart rate, control fatigue, and increase oxygen supply to the muscles, allowing you to perform at your best.

A simple mindful breathing practice during your S.I.T. workout can help you stay focused and calm. For example, as you perform high knees, consciously inhale and exhale in a steady rhythm, paying attention to the rise and fall of your chest. This focused breathing not only helps with endurance but also grounds you in the present moment.

B.Sensory awareness

Mindfulness encourages you to tune into the physical sensations of your body during exercise. When you perform each movement, notice how your muscles are engaging, how your joints are moving, and how your body feels as it works. This heightened sensory awareness helps you make adjustments to your technique, prevents injury, and allows you to fine-tune your performance.

For instance, as you move through squats or lunges, pay attention to the feeling of your legs working, the stretch in your hip flexors, and the engagement of your core. With each exercise, be aware of your body's alignment and how each muscle is activated. This awareness can make your workout more effective and enjoyable, as you're not just going through the motions but truly connecting with your body.

C.Reducing stress and anxiety

Mindfulness has long been associated with reducing stress and anxiety. Applying mindfulness to your workouts can provide a calming effect, helping you manage mental stress while improving physical health. During a S.I.T. workout, focusing on your body's movements and breath can help you manage the mental chatter that often arises in moments of physical intensity.

As your body works harder, your mind might become flooded with negative thoughts or worries. By practicing mindfulness, you can redirect your attention from those anxious thoughts and instead focus on the task at hand. This creates a sense of peace and clarity, reducing anxiety and allowing you to be more in control of your emotions during exercise.

3.The power of visualization

Visualization is another powerful tool that enhances mental focus during a workout. Visualization involves creating a mental image of success, progress, or the completion of your goals. In the context of your S.I.T. workout, you can visualize yourself completing each exercise with perfect form, feeling strong, and pushing through the intensity. This mental imagery can increase motivation, boost confidence, and even improve physical performance.

Before starting your workout, take a moment to visualize yourself completing the exercises. Imagine the movements, the muscles working, and the sense of accomplishment that comes with finishing the workout. Visualization helps set a positive tone and primes your mind for success. By mentally rehearsing your workout, you are preparing yourself for both the physical and mental challenges that lie ahead.

4.Developing a mind-body connection

Mindfulness and mental focus in training help cultivate a stronger mind-body connection, which is vital for overall fitness progress. The more in tune you are with how your body moves and responds during exercise, the more efficiently you can improve strength, flexibility, and endurance.

The mind-body connection is a powerful tool that allows you to make conscious adjustments during your workouts. For example, if you feel your form slipping during a push-up or plank, being mindful will allow you to correct it before injury occurs. This heightened awareness creates a more intentional workout, ensuring that every movement serves your fitness goals.

5.How to integrate focus and mindfulness into your S.I.T. routine

To begin incorporating mental focus and mindfulness into your S.I.T. workouts, here are some practical tips:

1.Start with breath awareness: Begin each workout by taking a few deep breaths, bringing your attention to your breath. Focus on slow, deliberate inhales and exhales to center yourself and reduce pre-workout jitters.

2.Set intentions: Before each set or exercise, set a clear intention. It could be focusing on maintaining perfect form, pushing through fatigue, or simply staying present throughout the workout. Setting an intention helps create a purpose behind each movement.

3.Stay present: Throughout the workout, constantly remind yourself to stay present. If your mind starts to wander, gently bring your focus back to the exercise and your breath. Be mindful of your body's sensations and avoid multitasking during your workout.

4.Visualize success: Take a moment to visualize completing each exercise with ease. Use positive mental imagery to enhance your belief in your abilities.

5.Reflect after the workout: Once you've finished your 7-minute S.I.T. workout, take a few moments to reflect. How did you feel during the workout? Were there any challenges you overcame? Practicing post-workout mindfulness helps reinforce the connection between the mind and body.

6.Conclusion

Incorporating mental focus and mindfulness into your training is not just about improving performance—it's about creating a deeper connection between your mind and body. By practicing mindfulness, you can make your workouts more effective, enjoyable, and sustainable. Whether you're doing a 7-minute S.I.T. workout or any other form of exercise, mental focus and mindfulness will help you maximize your results, reduce stress, and build a stronger mind-body connection. The next time you step onto the mat or start your S.I.T. workout, remember that your mind is just as important as your body in achieving your fitness goals.

Chapter 24: Tracking and measuring progress

One of the key components of any successful fitness journey is tracking and measuring progress. Whether you're performing a 7-minute S.I.T. workout, engaging in a more traditional exercise routine, or working toward specific fitness goals, knowing where you stand and how far you've come is crucial for continued improvement. It's easy to get discouraged if you don't see immediate results, but regular tracking can help you understand that progress is often gradual and incremental. In this chapter, we will explore how to effectively track and measure progress during your S.I.T. workouts and fitness journey.

1.Why tracking progress matters

Tracking your progress serves as both a motivational tool and a guide for adjusting your workout routine. By consistently measuring key performance indicators (KPIs), such as strength, endurance, flexibility, and even body composition, you can make informed decisions about your workouts and ensure that you're always moving toward your goals. Here's why progress tracking is so important:

A.Motivation and accountability

One of the greatest benefits of tracking progress is the motivational boost it provides. There will be days when your energy is low, and you may feel like skipping your workout. Having tangible proof of your progress can help you push through those moments. Whether it's a note in your fitness journal, a graph of your workout times, or an app tracking your calories burned, seeing your improvements over time can ignite a renewed sense of dedication.

Additionally, tracking progress makes you more accountable. If you're trying to reach a specific goal, such as improving your stamina or losing weight, tracking makes it easier to stay focused and take actionable steps toward that goal.

B.Identifying patterns

Tracking helps you identify patterns in your performance. For example, if you consistently perform a particular exercise at a faster pace or with better form, you can observe that you're improving over time. This information is invaluable for determining what's working well and what might need tweaking in your routine. For instance, if your cardio endurance is improving but your strength is plateauing, you might decide to incorporate more strength-focused exercises into your next S.I.T. workout.

C.Adjusting for continued growth

Measuring progress allows you to assess whether your current workout routine is pushing you enough. If you're improving too slowly, you can increase the intensity of your exercises or try new variations to stimulate progress. Conversely, if you feel your body is not recovering properly, tracking can highlight areas where you might need more rest or variety to avoid overtraining.

By measuring different aspects of your fitness regularly, you can continuously fine-tune your approach to ensure long-term growth and avoid hitting a plateau.

2.Key metrics to track

When it comes to tracking progress, there are many factors you can measure. These measurements not only help you track improvements but also offer valuable insights into your overall fitness level. Below are the key metrics you should consider tracking during your S.I.T. workouts.

A.Workout duration and intensity

One of the simplest ways to track progress in your S.I.T. workouts is by measuring the time it takes you to complete the routine. Initially, you may find that you're struggling to complete the full 7 minutes without breaks, but over time, your endurance will improve, and you'll be able to push through the entire workout with less effort.

You can also measure intensity by noting how hard each workout feels. The Borg Rating of Perceived Exertion (RPE) scale, for example, asks you to rate your workout intensity on a scale of 1 to 10, with 1 being very light activity and 10 being maximum effort. Tracking how your RPE improves over time helps gauge the effectiveness of your workouts and ensures that you're consistently challenging yourself.

B.Exercise performance

Within the S.I.T. workout, you perform a variety of exercises such as burpees, push-ups, squats, mountain climbers, and jumping jacks. Tracking the number of reps or sets completed for each exercise can provide insight into your strength, endurance, and power. For example, if you initially struggle to perform 10 push-ups but gradually increase to 20 or more, this demonstrates significant improvement in upper body strength.

Additionally, note how your form improves. Better form equals more effective workouts and fewer injuries. If you feel stronger, more stable, or capable of increasing the number of repetitions, it's a sure sign that you're making progress.

C.Heart rate and recovery time

Tracking your heart rate during and after your S.I.T. workout provides an excellent indication of your cardiovascular fitness. During high-intensity exercises, your heart rate should elevate significantly, and it should gradually return to normal during the rest periods. Over time, you should notice that your recovery time decreases—the time it takes for your heart rate to return to a resting state becomes shorter as your fitness improves. This is a key marker of cardiovascular health and overall fitness.

You can track your heart rate using a fitness tracker, smart watch, or manual pulse checks. Monitoring heart rate variability can provide more advanced insights into your recovery and general fitness levels.

D.Flexibility and mobility

Although S.I.T. workouts primarily focus on strength and cardiovascular fitness, flexibility and mobility also play a role in overall fitness. Tracking your flexibility—such as how far you can stretch in exercises like forward bends, lunges, or even hip openers—can help you assess improvements in range of motion. As your muscles become stronger and more conditioned through regular exercise, they should also become more flexible.

For example, you may find that you can squat lower or move through lunges with greater ease as you develop better mobility. Tracking these small changes can help prevent injuries by ensuring that your muscles and joints remain flexible and functional.

E.Body composition

While weight alone is not always the best indicator of fitness progress, tracking changes in body composition can provide a much clearer picture. Body composition refers to the proportion of fat, muscle, and bone in your body. As you continue your S.I.T. workouts, you may notice that you are gaining muscle while losing fat, leading to a leaner physique.

Regular body measurements—such as waist circumference, body fat percentage, or muscle mass—can help you assess these changes. If your goal is weight loss, tracking fat loss specifically (as opposed to overall weight) is crucial to understanding the effectiveness of your workout routine.

You can use skinfold calipers, bioelectrical impedance devices, or body composition scales to monitor changes in your body composition.

3.Tools for tracking progress

Now that you know which metrics to track, it's important to choose the right tools for the job. Here are some methods and tools you can use to measure and record your progress.

A.Fitness apps

There are a variety of fitness apps that can help you track your S.I.T. workouts, set goals, and monitor improvements. Popular apps like MyFitnessPal, Fitbit, and Strava allow you to log your workouts, track heart rate, set goals, and record body measurements. These apps provide easy-to-use interfaces, charts, and reports that can help you stay on top of your progress.

B.Fitness journals

If you prefer a more hands-on approach, a fitness journal can be a great tool for tracking your progress. Writing down your workouts, the exercises performed, and the number of sets or reps can help you stay focused on your goals. Additionally, tracking how you feel after each workout and noting any improvements in strength or endurance can provide valuable insight over time.

C.Wearable fitness trackers

Wearable fitness trackers such as the Apple Watch, Garmin, or Polar heart rate monitors can help you monitor your heart rate, calories burned, and recovery times. These devices also allow you to set fitness goals and receive notifications when you hit milestones. Wearables also track steps, sleep quality, and overall activity, making them great all-around tools for measuring fitness progress.

4.How to use your progress data

Once you've started tracking your progress, it's essential to use the data to guide your training. For instance, if you notice that your strength and endurance have plateaued, it may be time to increase the intensity of your workouts, adjust the exercises, or add new challenges. On the other hand, if you're consistently improving your heart rate recovery or completing more repetitions, you can celebrate those successes and stay motivated to keep going.

5.Conclusion

Tracking and measuring progress is one of the most powerful tools you have in your fitness journey. Whether you're training with S.I.T., running, or focusing on weightlifting, measuring key metrics such as workout duration, intensity, exercise performance, heart rate, and body composition can help you stay focused, motivated, and committed to your goals. Regularly tracking your progress gives you the data you need to make informed decisions about your workouts and ensures that you're continually pushing toward new heights in your fitness journey.

Chapter 25: Group training at home

Group training is a fantastic way to stay motivated, improve performance, and foster a sense of community while working toward fitness goals. However, the idea of group training is often associated with large gyms or fitness centers, where people gather in person for classes. The concept of group training doesn't have to be confined to the gym; in fact, group training at home can be just as effective and even more convenient. Whether you're looking to create your own fitness community or join a virtual one, home group training can offer many benefits—both physically and mentally. In this chapter, we will explore the many advantages of group training at home, how to set it up, and how to stay motivated in a group training environment.

1.The benefits of group training at home

Training with others can significantly enhance your workout experience, offering a wide range of benefits that support both physical and mental well-being. Group training brings an extra layer of motivation, accountability, and fun, which can be hard to achieve when exercising alone. Here's a closer look at why group training at home is such a powerful tool:

A.Motivation and accountability

One of the main benefits of group training is the motivation it provides. When you're training in a group, you're more likely to push yourself harder than when you work out alone. This is because you draw inspiration from those around you, whether it's through friendly competition, encouragement, or simply the collective energy of the group.

At home, accountability plays a crucial role. Whether you're part of an online workout community or simply training with family or friends, knowing that others are depending on you to show up can help you stay committed to your fitness routine. When the workout is scheduled with others, you're less likely to hit the snooze button or skip the session altogether.

B.Social connection

In a time where many people are working from home or spending more time isolated, group training can serve as an important source of social connection. Fitness isn't just about physical strength; it's also about building relationships and sharing experiences. Whether you're meeting online through a video call or working out with a friend in your living room, the camaraderie that group training provides is one of the key ingredients for long-term success.

The sense of community created during group training can also boost your mental health. Interacting with others while working toward common fitness goals helps create bonds and build relationships, fostering a positive and supportive environment.

C.Fun and variety

Group training injects an element of fun into your workouts, which is often difficult to achieve when you're exercising alone. Different people bring their unique energy to a group, and workouts tend to be more dynamic and lively in a group setting. The excitement of having multiple people participating can motivate you to push through fatigue and make the workout experience enjoyable.

Additionally, group workouts often include different types of exercises, which can add variety to your routine. This variety helps keep things interesting and prevents you from getting bored or falling into a fitness plateau. The diversity in exercises can also be great for improving overall fitness, as you'll likely work on different muscle groups and move in new ways.

D.Encouragement and support

In a group setting, encouragement is readily available. It's not uncommon for participants to cheer each other on, offer positive reinforcement, or share tips on form and technique. This encouragement is particularly beneficial for beginners, who may feel nervous or intimidated about exercising. Having a supportive group helps to boost confidence, creating an atmosphere where everyone can feel comfortable and motivated to improve.

Whether you're tackling a challenging exercise or pushing through a particularly intense interval, hearing positive affirmations from the group can help you stay focused and motivated to complete the session.

2.How to set up group training at home

Creating a group training environment at home doesn't have to be complicated. With the right approach, it can be seamless, effective, and fun. Here are some key steps to help you get started:

A.Choose the right platform or space

Whether you want to connect with friends or join a virtual fitness group, you'll need a space and platform that works for everyone involved. For virtual group training, apps like Zoom, Skype, or Google Meet can be great platforms for connecting with others and following along in real-time. These platforms offer video and audio features, allowing you to communicate with your group and receive live feedback from the instructor or fellow participants.

If you're hosting group training in person, create a designated workout space in your home where everyone can move freely and safely. Ideally, this space should be free of obstacles, with enough room for exercises like jumping jacks, lunges, or squats. Make sure the area is well-lit and well-ventilated to ensure everyone is comfortable during the workout.

B.Select a suitable workout program

Group training is most effective when everyone follows a structured workout program. Since you'll be working out at home, it's important to choose a program that can be performed in a limited space and without complicated equipment. The 7-minute S.I.T. workout is a perfect example of a time-efficient, space-friendly workout that can be done in a group setting. You can perform a variety of exercises like burpees, push-ups, mountain climbers, and jumping jacks, all in the comfort of your own home.

If you have access to equipment, you could incorporate dumbbells, resistance bands, or kettlebells for added intensity, but you don't need these to make your workout effective. Alternatively, you can use an app that offers group workouts, such as a virtual HIIT class or a fitness challenge.

C.Set clear goals and expectations

Before starting your group workout, set clear expectations about the goals and objectives of the training session. Are you aiming to improve strength, endurance, or cardiovascular fitness? Is the goal to have fun, challenge each other, or compete? Communicating these objectives will help everyone in the group stay on track and ensure that everyone gets the most out of the session.

If you're training with friends or family, it's important to establish a workout schedule that works for everyone. Whether you meet once a week or have daily sessions, consistency is key. Having a set time for your group workouts will help keep everyone committed.

D.Provide encouragement and feedback

A key component of group training is support and feedback. During a group session, encourage your fellow participants by cheering them on or offering positive reinforcement. If you're leading the session, make sure to give constructive feedback on form and technique while also celebrating individual achievements.

Don't forget to keep things lighthearted and fun. Group training is about building a supportive community, so fostering a positive, inclusive environment will help everyone feel comfortable and motivated to keep going.

3.Types of group training you can do at home

There are many different types of group workouts you can do at home. The beauty of training at home is that you can be creative with your approach. Here are a few ideas for types of group workouts that work well in a home setting:

A.Virtual group classes

If you're looking for structure and guidance, you can sign up for online fitness classes that are streamed live. Many trainers and fitness studios offer group training sessions via platforms like Zoom or YouTube. These can range from yoga and Pilates to HIIT and strength training. Group members can participate from anywhere and still feel like part of a team.

B.Partner workouts

Partner workouts are a fun way to bond while getting fit. You and a friend or family member can perform exercises that involve teamwork, like partner push-ups, medicine ball tosses, or high-fives during planks. Working in pairs also adds a competitive element, which can help keep the energy high.

C.Challenges and competitions

You can also organize fitness challenges with your group, such as who can perform the most burpees in one minute, hold a plank for the longest time, or complete the most rounds of a particular workout in seven minutes. These friendly competitions can add an element of fun and push everyone to give their best effort.

D.Circuit workouts

Create a circuit of different exercises that participants can rotate through. For example, you could set up five stations: squats, push-ups, mountain climbers, jumping jacks, and planks. Each person performs a set amount of reps at each station before moving on to the next. Circuits are a great way to keep the workout varied and allow each participant to focus on different exercises throughout the session.

4.Staying motivated in group training

Maintaining motivation during group training at home is key to ensuring consistency and success. Here are some tips to stay motivated:

1.Create a group chat: Having a communication channel like a group chat allows everyone to stay connected between workouts, share progress, and encourage each other. Sharing accomplishments, struggles, and tips in real-time can help keep motivation levels high.

2.Celebrate milestones: Make sure to celebrate milestones, whether it's reaching a fitness goal, improving your workout time, or simply completing a challenging session. Acknowledge each person's progress to keep the group spirit alive.

3.Set group goals: Group goals—such as completing a certain number of workouts or achieving a collective fitness milestone—can provide a sense of camaraderie and encourage everyone to work together toward a common objective.

4.Mix it up: To keep everyone engaged, switch up the workouts regularly. Introduce new exercises, change the order of the routine, or set new challenges to avoid monotony.

5.Conclusion

Group training at home is a powerful way to stay motivated, build social connections, and achieve your fitness goals. Whether you're working out with family, friends, or joining an online fitness community, group training creates a sense of accountability, support, and fun that is hard to replicate when training solo. By choosing the right workouts, setting clear goals, and fostering a positive environment, you can make group training at home a rewarding and enjoyable experience that enhances both your physical and mental well-being.

Chapter 26: Common mistakes and how to avoid them

Embarking on a fitness journey can be an exciting and rewarding experience, especially when following a structured workout program like the 7-minute S.I.T. workout. However, as with any fitness routine, mistakes can arise along the way. Whether you're new to working out or have been exercising for a while, it's important to recognize common pitfalls and learn how to avoid them to ensure that you stay on track and achieve your fitness goals effectively. In this chapter, we will identify some of the most common mistakes people make when doing home workouts and provide practical tips for avoiding them.

1.Skipping warm-up and cool-down

Mistake:

One of the most frequent mistakes made by individuals when doing the 7-minute S.I.T. workout or any other fitness routine is neglecting the warm-up and cool-down phases. Many people are eager to jump right into the workout, especially when time is limited, and they underestimate the importance of preparing the body before exercising and allowing it to recover afterward.

How to avoid It:

A proper warm-up prepares your body for physical activity by increasing blood flow to your muscles, enhancing joint mobility, and reducing the risk of injury. A good warm-up should last about 5 to 10 minutes and include dynamic movements like leg swings, arm circles, and gentle cardio exercises such as jogging in place or jumping jacks.

Similarly, cooling down after a workout allows your heart rate to gradually return to normal, prevents dizziness, and promotes muscle recovery. Stretching and deep breathing exercises during the cool-down phase help reduce muscle tightness and improve flexibility.

Incorporating both warm-up and cool-down into your workout routine may take a little extra time, but it will help you avoid injuries and improve your overall performance.

2.Poor form and technique

Mistake:

Another common mistake is performing exercises with improper form or technique. This is especially true for bodyweight exercises like squats, push-ups, and burpees, where the risk of injury is high if movements are not executed correctly. Poor form can lead to strain on your joints, back, and muscles, reducing the effectiveness of your workout and increasing the chances of injury.

How to avoid It:

Focus on learning the correct technique for each exercise before increasing the intensity or volume. Whether you're doing push-ups, squats, or planks, ensure that your body is aligned properly to avoid unnecessary stress on your joints.

For example, during a squat, make sure your knees don't extend beyond your toes, and your weight is shifted onto your heels. In a push-up, keep your body in a straight line from your head to your heels, and engage your core to avoid sagging in your lower back. If you're unsure about your form, consider recording your exercises and reviewing them to spot any errors, or seek guidance from a qualified fitness professional.

To make sure you're progressing safely, slow down your movements if necessary and perform fewer repetitions at first to perfect your form. As your technique improves, you can gradually increase the intensity.

3.Overtraining and insufficient rest

Mistake:

Many individuals, especially those who are new to fitness or are eager to achieve quick results, tend to overtrain. They push themselves too hard, too often, without allowing enough time for their body to recover. Overtraining can lead to fatigue, diminished performance, and an increased risk of injury.

How to avoid It:

While consistency is essential for progress, so is rest. Your body needs time to recover between workouts to repair muscles, replenish energy stores, and reduce the risk of injury. For the 7-minute S.I.T. workout, which is an intense burst of exercise, it's important to follow a well-balanced routine that includes rest days or active recovery days.

A general rule of thumb is to schedule at least one or two rest days per week, depending on your fitness level. Active recovery activities such as walking, yoga, or light stretching can also help keep your body moving without overtaxing it.

Pay attention to how your body feels during and after workouts. If you're experiencing persistent soreness, fatigue, or joint pain, it may be a sign that you're overtraining and need more rest.

4.Neglecting nutrition and hydration

Mistake:

Exercise alone is not enough to achieve optimal fitness results. Many people neglect the importance of nutrition and hydration, which play a critical role in fueling the body for exercise, enhancing performance, and aiding recovery. Inadequate nutrition and dehydration can lead to fatigue, poor performance, and slower recovery times.

How to avoid It:

Make sure you're eating a balanced diet that supports your fitness goals. Focus on consuming nutrient-dense foods such as fruits, vegetables, lean proteins, whole grains, and healthy fats. Prioritize protein intake to support muscle recovery and growth, especially after intense workouts like S.I.T.

Hydration is just as important. Make sure to drink water before, during, and after your workouts to stay hydrated and support optimal performance. Dehydration can lead to muscle cramps, fatigue, and decreased endurance, so aim to drink enough water throughout the day, especially if you're exercising regularly.

If you're unsure about your nutrition needs, consider consulting a nutritionist to develop a meal plan that aligns with your goals.

5.Doing the same routine every day

Mistake:

Sticking to the same workout routine day after day can quickly lead to boredom, plateaus, and diminished results. While consistency is important, doing the same exercises every day doesn't challenge your body enough to keep progressing. The body adapts to repetitive routines, which can prevent further gains in strength, endurance, or muscle tone.

How to avoid It:

Variety is key in any workout routine. The 7-minute S.I.T. workout itself offers a variety of exercises, but you can take it a step further by changing up your routine every few weeks. Try incorporating different bodyweight exercises, adding resistance, or adjusting the intensity level to keep your workouts fresh and challenging.

You can also experiment with different types of workouts, such as HIIT, yoga, Pilates, or strength training, to complement your S.I.T. routine. Adding variety not only helps you break through plateaus but also keeps your workouts interesting and enjoyable.

6.Setting unrealistic goals

Mistake:

Setting overly ambitious goals that are not achievable within a reasonable time frame is another mistake that can derail your fitness journey. While having goals is essential, it's important to set goals that are specific, measurable, and realistic. Unrealistic expectations can lead to frustration, burnout, and even injury when you push yourself too hard.

How to avoid It:

Set small, incremental goals that align with your fitness level and progress. For example, instead of aiming to lose 20 pounds in a month, focus on achieving small goals such as completing your workouts consistently for a week, improving your endurance, or increasing your strength. Track your progress regularly and celebrate your successes, no matter how small they may seem.

Using SMART (Specific, Measurable, Achievable, Relevant, and Time-bound) goals is a helpful strategy to ensure that your objectives are realistic and achievable.

7.Ignoring mental health and rest

Mistake:

Exercise is great for physical health, but it's important not to neglect your mental health in the process. Many people focus solely on physical performance and body aesthetics, but mental well-being plays an equally important role in your fitness journey. Ignoring your mental health can lead to stress, burnout, and a lack of motivation.

How to avoid It:

Incorporate mindfulness practices into your routine, such as meditation, deep breathing exercises, or journaling, to support your mental well-being. Remember that fitness is not just about physical results but also about feeling good mentally. Rest and recovery aren't just for your body—they're essential for maintaining a healthy mind as well.

Conclusion

Fitness is a journey, not a destination, and along the way, it's easy to make mistakes. By avoiding common pitfalls such as skipping warm-ups, neglecting form, overtraining, or setting unrealistic goals, you can ensure that your workouts are effective, safe, and sustainable. Remember, the key to success is consistency, progress, and learning from your mistakes. Keep an open mind, listen to your body, and continue refining your approach as you grow stronger, healthier, and more fit.

Chapter 27: Combining S.I.T. with ther workouts

One of the greatest aspects of the 7-minute S.I.T. (Speed Interval Training) workout is its versatility. It's efficient, effective, and easily adaptable to various fitness levels and goals. While the S.I.T. workout is a powerful standalone routine, combining it with other workout types can offer a comprehensive approach to fitness, helping you achieve a well-rounded, balanced training plan. Whether you are looking to improve strength, increase cardiovascular fitness, enhance flexibility, or focus on specific muscle groups, integrating different forms of exercise with S.I.T. can help you maximize your fitness results. In this chapter, we'll explore how combining S.I.T. with other workouts can enhance your overall fitness journey.

1.The benefits of combining S.I.T. with other workouts

A.Balanced fitness development

Although S.I.T. workouts are incredibly effective for building cardiovascular endurance, stamina, and overall body conditioning, they mainly focus on high-intensity intervals and bodyweight exercises. While this provides great results for general fitness, it may not fully target every muscle group or develop other important fitness components, such as strength, flexibility, or mobility. By pairing S.I.T. with other workout types, you can address these gaps and create a balanced workout routine.

For example, while S.I.T. may focus on explosiveness, incorporating strength training into your routine will enhance muscle development and promote overall power. Similarly, flexibility exercises like yoga or Pilates can help you increase mobility, improve posture, and prevent injury.

B.Increased motivation and variety

One of the challenges people face when sticking to a workout routine is boredom. Doing the same exercises repeatedly can make your workouts feel monotonous, which can lead to a lack of motivation. Mixing up your workout plan by combining S.I.T. with other types of exercises can keep things fresh, exciting, and enjoyable.

In addition, alternating between different workout styles helps target different aspects of fitness, which can lead to better overall progress. Variety prevents plateaus, and the excitement of trying new exercises can keep you motivated and focused on your goals.

C.More efficient results

Combining different types of workouts allows you to maximize your efforts in a shorter amount of time. For example, while S.I.T. targets your cardiovascular fitness and endurance, strength training works on muscle mass and fat loss. By incorporating both into your routine, you're optimizing your time, working multiple components of fitness simultaneously, and seeing better results in less time.

By focusing on the most efficient methods for each area of fitness, you're ensuring that you're improving your overall fitness level, not just one component.

2.How to combine S.I.T. with strength training

A.S.I.T. + strength training for muscle and fat loss

Strength training is essential for building lean muscle, increasing metabolism, and improving overall strength. Combining S.I.T. with weightlifting or resistance training is an excellent way to improve your strength and endurance simultaneously.

The key to combining these two is finding the right balance. S.I.T. focuses on short bursts of high-intensity cardio, while strength training involves lifting weights or using resistance to target specific muscle groups. The ideal combination would involve alternating between the two, ensuring that your body gets the benefits of both without overexertion.

For example, on one day, you could perform a full-body S.I.T. workout followed by a 20-minute strength training session focusing on upper body exercises like push-ups, dumbbell rows, and shoulder presses. On another day, you could focus on lower body strength with squats, lunges, and deadlifts, followed by a shorter but intense S.I.T. session.

B.Using circuit training

Circuit training combines both cardio and strength training in a single workout, making it a perfect method for pairing with S.I.T. During a circuit workout, you can alternate between strength exercises and high-intensity intervals. For instance, a circuit could include 30 seconds of squats (strength) followed by 30 seconds of jumping jacks (cardio) and then 30 seconds of dumbbell curls (strength), and repeat.

This type of circuit workout combines the benefits of both strength training and cardiovascular fitness, improving endurance and muscle tone. The intensity of the S.I.T. intervals will elevate your heart rate while strength exercises build muscle and promote fat loss. This approach ensures that both strength and cardio are equally emphasized.

3.Combining S.I.T. with flexibility and mobility work

A.S.I.T. + yoga or pilates for flexibility

S.I.T. workouts are great for improving cardiovascular health and boosting overall fitness. However, S.I.T. primarily focuses on explosive movements and strength endurance, which may lead to muscle tightness or reduced flexibility if not counterbalanced with stretching or mobility work.

Incorporating yoga or Pilates into your routine can significantly improve your flexibility, mobility, and posture. Yoga, in particular, helps with joint health, flexibility, and mental relaxation. Pilates focuses on core strength and stability, which is especially beneficial after doing intense movements in S.I.T.

After completing your S.I.T. workout, a 10-15 minute yoga session can stretch and lengthen the muscles worked, aiding in recovery. Some poses that work well after S.I.T. include downward dog, cobra, and pigeon pose, which target the hamstrings, lower back, and hip flexors. Pilates exercises like the "swimming" move or "the hundred" help to build core strength and stability, balancing out the dynamic movements in S.I.T.

B.Active recovery days with yoga or stretching

On your rest days, consider incorporating yoga or a stretching routine to maintain flexibility and prevent muscle tightness. Active recovery can enhance recovery, improve mobility, and prevent injuries, ensuring that your body is ready for the next round of high-intensity workouts. Stretching can also be beneficial in alleviating soreness caused by intense S.I.T. workouts, helping you feel more refreshed and less stiff.

4.Combining S.I.T. with endurance training

A.S.I.T. + running or cycling for cardiovascular fitness

While S.I.T. is great for improving cardiovascular fitness, adding longer endurance workouts like running or cycling into your routine can help build stamina, enhance aerobic capacity, and improve heart health. These activities are lower in intensity than S.I.T. but are great for building endurance over time.

To combine S.I.T. with endurance training, alternate between high-intensity intervals and steady-state cardio. For example, on one day, you could do a 7-minute S.I.T. session to work on explosiveness and stamina, followed by a 30-minute steady run or bike ride at a moderate pace to build endurance.

On other days, you might opt for a 30-minute cycling session followed by a shorter, high-intensity S.I.T. workout targeting specific muscle groups, such as core exercises or bodyweight squats. This blend of short bursts and longer cardio efforts will ensure you're improving both speed and stamina, making your cardiovascular fitness well-rounded.

5.Combining S.I.T. with HIIT

A.S.I.T. + traditional HIIT for increased intensity

S.I.T. is, in essence, a form of high-intensity interval training (HIIT), but it is typically shorter and focuses on bodyweight exercises. If you're looking to take your workouts to the next level, combining traditional HIIT with S.I.T. can provide an even greater intensity boost, accelerating fat loss, building endurance, and increasing strength.

Traditional HIIT may involve more varied exercises, including weightlifting, plyometric moves, or sprints. For example, you could alternate between 30 seconds of intense sprinting (HIIT) and 30 seconds of bodyweight exercises like burpees or high knees (S.I.T.). This combination will push your cardiovascular endurance to new heights and challenge your muscles in different ways.

By adding more challenging movements like kettlebell swings, jump squats, or battle ropes into your routine, you'll engage more muscle groups and promote greater caloric burn and muscle endurance. HIIT sessions typically last anywhere from 15 to 30 minutes, so you can alternate between these longer HIIT intervals and shorter S.I.T. workouts, maximizing your calorie burn and fitness gains.

6.Structuring a balanced weekly workout plan

To achieve a comprehensive fitness routine, you can structure your week by combining S.I.T. with different types of workouts, ensuring that you're targeting multiple fitness components while allowing adequate recovery time.

Example weekly plan:

- **Monday:** S.I.T. workout + Strength training (upper body)
- **Tuesday:** Yoga or Pilates for flexibility + Light cardio
- **Wednesday:** S.I.T. workout + Strength training (lower body)
- **Thursday:** Active recovery or rest day
- **Friday:** Long endurance cardio (running/cycling) + S.I.T. workout
- **Saturday:** Full-body strength training circuit + Light yoga/stretching
- **Sunday:** Rest day or gentle yoga for recovery

This schedule allows you to alternate between intense S.I.T. workouts, strength training, cardio, and flexibility work, ensuring that all aspects of fitness are addressed throughout the week.

Conclusion

Combining the 7-minute S.I.T. workout with other types of exercise is a powerful way to optimize your fitness and keep your routine exciting. Whether you pair S.I.T. with strength training, flexibility exercises, or endurance training, you'll be creating a balanced and effective program that addresses every component of fitness. By maintaining variety, you'll also prevent plateaus, keep your motivation high, and achieve more well-rounded results.

Chapter 28: The role of music and rhythm

The connection between exercise and music is not a new concept. For decades, athletes and fitness enthusiasts alike have been turning to music as a tool to enhance their workouts. Whether it's lifting weights, running, or participating in high-intensity workouts like the 7-minute S.I.T. workout, music can serve as both a motivator and a guide, helping individuals push through fatigue and maintain focus. The power of rhythm and sound in training goes beyond simple enjoyment; it taps into the psychological and physiological aspects of exercise, improving performance, mood, and overall workout efficiency.

In this chapter, we'll explore the role of music and rhythm in workouts, focusing specifically on how it can impact your experience with S.I.T. workouts. We'll delve into the science behind why music works, how to choose the right playlist, and how rhythm can sync with high-intensity training to maximize results.

1.The psychological impact of music on exercise

A.Boosting motivation

The most immediate benefit of listening to music during a workout is its ability to boost motivation. Music has a unique ability to uplift and energize us, which is essential when performing physically demanding activities like S.I.T. workouts. A fast-paced, energetic playlist can ignite excitement and increase enthusiasm, making it easier to get started and stick with your workout routine.

Research has shown that music can distract the mind from feelings of discomfort or fatigue, especially during high-intensity intervals. As you power through those tough S.I.T. moments, the rhythm and beat of your playlist help to take your focus off the physical strain and reframe your perception of exertion. This distraction effect can make challenging exercises feel more manageable, encouraging individuals to push beyond their limits.

B.Enhancing mood and reducing stress

Another psychological benefit of listening to music during exercise is its impact on mood and stress levels. High-intensity workouts like S.I.T. often create physical stress on the body, and music can serve as a mental tool to counterbalance this. It can create a sense of enjoyment, positivity, and fun, which can reduce the perception of stress and anxiety associated with tough workouts.

When engaging in intense physical activities, such as the 7-minute S.I.T. workout, your body produces endorphins—the brain's "feel-good" chemicals. Music can stimulate this release of endorphins, intensifying the mood-boosting effects of exercise and helping you feel more energized and motivated throughout your session. Whether you're working out at home or at the gym, the right tunes can help you stay positive and relaxed, preventing frustration or negative thoughts that could derail your performance.

2.The physiological effects of music on performance

A.Synchronization with movements

Rhythm plays a significant role in how music affects our physical performance. The synchronization of music with movement is a technique known as "entrainment," where your body subconsciously aligns its movements with the beat of the music. In high-intensity interval training, this synchronization can improve timing and coordination, allowing you to execute exercises more efficiently and fluidly.

For example, in the 7-minute S.I.T. workout, the rhythm of the music can guide your movements, particularly during exercises like jumping jacks, burpees, or mountain climbers. A fast tempo can encourage quick, explosive movements, while a slower beat might be more appropriate for cooldown exercises. Research suggests that matching your exercise tempo with a song's rhythm can lead to improved coordination, making it easier to maintain consistent effort throughout each interval.

B.Increased physical endurance

Music also plays a key role in increasing physical endurance. Studies have shown that people who listen to music during exercise tend to perform better and experience less perceived exertion than those who work out in silence. The energizing effect of music can help you maintain a high level of intensity during a S.I.T. workout, which requires bursts of effort followed by short recovery periods.

The rhythmic structure of music can also aid in regulating pacing. When doing high-intensity intervals, it's easy to overexert yourself in the beginning or lose energy toward the end. Music with a consistent tempo can help regulate your pacing, ensuring that you maintain a steady, sustainable effort throughout the entire session. This can be especially important when working at maximum effort during the high-intensity phases of S.I.T. workouts.

3.The science of music and exercise

A.Cognitive benefits of music

The cognitive effects of music on exercise are closely tied to motivation, focus, and attention. During high-intensity training like S.I.T., it's easy for your mind to wander, which may lead to a decrease in focus and performance. Music serves as an external focus point, allowing you to concentrate on the rhythm and beat rather than fatigue or discomfort.

Research also suggests that listening to music can improve cognitive performance during exercise by enhancing concentration and task performance. In the case of a 7-minute S.I.T. workout, where the exercise duration is relatively short but intense, music can help you stay in the zone, allowing you to maintain a higher level of focus and intensity throughout each exercise.

B.Reducing perception of fatigue

One of the most significant psychological benefits of music is its ability to reduce the perception of fatigue. During a high-intensity workout like S.I.T., your muscles may begin to feel fatigued, and your heart rate will rise, signaling to your brain that it's time to slow down. However, music helps mask these signals by diverting your attention, which reduces the sensation of exhaustion.

The tempo, rhythm, and volume of the music can also play a role in how fatigue is perceived. Faster tempos and louder volumes tend to provide more energy and reduce the perception of effort, while slower tempos may have a calming effect, which is beneficial during recovery periods or cooldown.

4.How to choose the right music for S.I.T. workouts

A.Tempo and intensity

When selecting music for your S.I.T. workout, tempo is crucial. Upbeat, high-energy songs with a fast tempo—typically ranging between 120 to 160 beats per minute (BPM)—are ideal for high-intensity interval training. These fast tempos align with the explosive movements performed during S.I.T. exercises, helping to maintain a high pace and keep you energized throughout each interval.

For example, electronic dance music (EDM), hip-hop, or fast rock songs often provide the quick tempo needed for an intense workout. Songs with a driving beat can push you to keep moving at a quick pace, ensuring that you stay motivated and energized during each high-intensity segment.

During the rest or cooldown intervals, consider switching to slower, more relaxing music with a lower BPM, around 60 to 90 BPM. This will help you relax, reduce your heart rate, and improve your recovery. Soft instrumental music, acoustic tracks, or even classical music can help ease your body back into a state of rest and relaxation.

B.Lyrics vs. instrumental music

The choice between music with lyrics and instrumental music can depend on personal preference. Some people find that songs with lyrics can enhance motivation, especially if the lyrics are uplifting or align with the workout's energy. However, others may find lyrics distracting, particularly during high-intensity workouts when focus is essential.

If you find lyrics distracting, instrumental music such as electronic beats, classical music, or ambient tunes can help you stay focused on the workout without the added mental load of following words. Ultimately, the choice between instrumental or lyrical music comes down to what helps you maintain the best flow during your workout.

5.Music and rhythm in group workouts

A.Social and group dynamics

While music is often associated with individual workouts, it also plays a significant role in group training sessions. In a group setting, music can unite participants by creating a shared rhythm and energy. The collective experience of working out to the same beat enhances social cohesion, making the workout feel more fun and motivating.

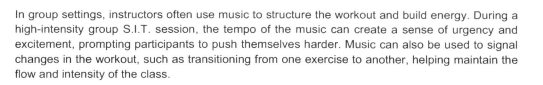

In group settings, instructors often use music to structure the workout and build energy. During a high-intensity group S.I.T. session, the tempo of the music can create a sense of urgency and excitement, prompting participants to push themselves harder. Music can also be used to signal changes in the workout, such as transitioning from one exercise to another, helping maintain the flow and intensity of the class.

Conclusion

The role of music and rhythm in a 7-minute S.I.T. workout is much more than just background noise. It serves as a powerful motivator, cognitive enhancer, and physical performance booster. The right music can energize you, reduce fatigue, and improve focus, making your high-intensity interval training more enjoyable and effective. Whether you're working out at home or in a group setting, music has the potential to elevate your fitness experience. By choosing the right tempo, energy, and rhythm to match your S.I.T. workouts, you can take your performance to new heights, making each session both mentally and physically rewarding.

Chapter 29: Success stories

When it comes to fitness, we all need motivation. Whether we're just starting out on our journey or have been working hard for years, hearing success stories can be the spark that ignites our own progress. The power of personal stories lies in their ability to inspire us to push through obstacles, stay committed, and believe in the possibility of transformation. This chapter will explore real-life success stories of individuals who have used the 7-minute S.I.T. workout to achieve incredible results, both physically and mentally.

These success stories are a testament to the efficiency and effectiveness of S.I.T. and highlight how small, consistent efforts can lead to significant changes in one's health, fitness, and overall well-being. Whether the goal is weight loss, strength building, improved cardiovascular fitness, or increased confidence, these stories demonstrate that with the right mindset, anyone can achieve their goals using the S.I.T. workout method.

1.Maria's weight loss journey: Shedding 30 pounds in 3 months

Maria, a busy professional and mother of two, struggled for years with her weight. She had tried several diets and exercise programs but found it difficult to stick with anything long-term due to her demanding schedule. Maria's turning point came when she discovered the 7-minute S.I.T. workout.

"I was skeptical at first," Maria recalls. "I thought, 'How could a 7-minute workout really make a difference? I need more time, more intensity!' But I was so wrong."

Maria decided to give S.I.T. a try after learning about its benefits for weight loss and fat burning. She started by dedicating just 7 minutes in the morning to the workout, using her living room as her workout space. Initially, it was tough. She struggled with certain exercises, especially the high-intensity intervals. But after a few weeks, she began to notice a difference. Not only did she feel stronger, but she also had more energy throughout the day.

Over the next three months, Maria gradually increased her S.I.T. sessions to twice daily. By incorporating healthier eating habits and maintaining consistency, she managed to lose 30 pounds. The S.I.T. workout helped her build endurance, and she started to notice changes in her body composition as well. What was once a difficult 7 minutes became a fulfilling, energizing part of her day.

"I never thought 7 minutes could change so much," Maria says. "I'm in the best shape I've ever been, and I have more energy to keep up with my kids and my job. The best part is that I can do it at home, which makes it so easy to stay consistent."

Maria's story is a powerful reminder that even short, intense workouts can lead to substantial weight loss results, especially when combined with healthy eating and dedication.

2.Jake's transformation: Building strength and confidence

Jake, a 35-year-old office worker, had always struggled with feeling weak and lacking energy. He had tried various gym routines but often found himself feeling intimidated by larger, more experienced gym-goers. After years of frustration, Jake stumbled upon the concept of the 7-minute S.I.T. workout during a casual search online.

"I was looking for something quick and efficient," Jake explains. "I wasn't ready to commit to long gym sessions, but I wanted to feel stronger and more confident."

He started with the basic 7-minute S.I.T. workout, initially struggling with certain movements like burpees and mountain climbers. However, instead of getting discouraged, he focused on improving his form and performance each day. Jake soon began noticing that not only was his strength increasing, but his energy levels were also soaring. The physical benefits of S.I.T. were clear: he felt stronger, more agile, and more capable of performing everyday tasks with ease.

After six months of consistent practice, Jake saw impressive physical results. He had built muscle in his arms and legs, lost fat around his midsection, and felt more confident in his own skin. But perhaps the most significant transformation was mental. Jake felt more focused and energized at work and had developed a mindset that allowed him to push through other challenges in life.

"My body is stronger, and my confidence is higher," Jake says. "S.I.T. gave me the strength I never thought I had, and I've learned that my body can do way more than I ever imagined."

Jake's story highlights the potential for strength-building through short, focused workouts. With dedication and perseverance, the S.I.T. workout helped him build not only physical strength but mental resilience as well.

3.Sarah's postpartum recovery: Reclaiming her fitness

Sarah, a 29-year-old mother of one, had always been active and healthy. However, after giving birth to her son, she found herself struggling to get back into shape. Postpartum recovery was challenging, and Sarah found it difficult to find time to exercise between caring for her newborn and managing household responsibilities.

"I had a lot of body image issues and just didn't feel like myself after having my son," Sarah recalls. "I was exhausted, and going to the gym seemed impossible with a newborn."

After hearing about the benefits of the 7-minute S.I.T. workout for busy moms, Sarah decided to give it a try. She started with one session a day, focusing on gentle modifications to accommodate her postpartum body. Sarah found the short duration of the workout to be ideal, as it allowed her to fit it into her busy schedule without overwhelming herself.

After several weeks, Sarah began to feel stronger and noticed that her energy levels were significantly higher. She also found that the S.I.T. workout was effective in toning her muscles and rebuilding her core strength. Although it took time and patience, Sarah was able to shed the baby weight and reclaim her fitness with consistency and dedication.

"Having just 7 minutes to myself every day made all the difference," Sarah says. "It gave me the time and energy I needed to take care of myself, which in turn helped me take care of my baby."

Sarah's success story is a beautiful example of how even new mothers can regain their strength and fitness by committing to short, intense workouts. The 7-minute S.I.T. workout provided her with a manageable way to reclaim her body after childbirth, offering both physical and emotional benefits.

4.Kevin's journey: Overcoming a sedentary lifestyle

Kevin, a 42-year-old office worker, had spent years living a sedentary lifestyle. Long hours sitting at a desk and poor eating habits had led to weight gain, fatigue, and an overall decline in health. He was ready for a change but found the idea of committing to long hours at the gym daunting.

"I was in bad shape," Kevin admits. "I knew I needed to do something, but I didn't have time to spend hours at the gym. The idea of 7 minutes sounded doable, so I thought I'd give it a shot."

Kevin started with the 7-minute S.I.T. workout as a way to get his body moving again. At first, the intensity of the exercises left him feeling exhausted, but he stuck with it. Over time, his endurance improved, and he was able to perform the exercises more effectively. He began feeling less fatigued throughout the day and noticed positive changes in his overall health.

After six months of consistent 7-minute workouts, Kevin had lost 25 pounds, improved his cardiovascular fitness, and felt more energetic. Most importantly, he felt empowered and proud of his ability to maintain a routine that fit his lifestyle.

"The 7-minute S.I.T. workout was a game-changer for me," Kevin says. "It fit into my life perfectly, and it was the catalyst I needed to take control of my health again."

Kevin's success story highlights how even those who lead a sedentary lifestyle can make dramatic changes in their health by committing to a simple yet effective exercise routine like S.I.T.

5.Conclusion: Inspiration for your own journey

The success stories of Maria, Jake, Sarah, and Kevin demonstrate that with dedication, consistency, and the right workout strategy, anyone can transform their body and mindset. Whether you're looking to lose weight, gain strength, improve endurance, or reclaim your health, the 7-minute S.I.T. workout offers a practical, effective solution. These stories prove that even small, focused efforts can lead to monumental changes, empowering you to reach your fitness goals and live a healthier, more fulfilling life.

No matter where you are in your fitness journey, remember that success is achievable. Just like these individuals, you have the power to transform your life—one 7-minute workout at a time. Stay motivated, stay committed, and your own success story may be just around the corner.

Chapter 30: Your personal training plan

Embarking on a fitness journey can often feel overwhelming, especially when you're trying to figure out the best plan for yourself. The key to success in any fitness regimen is not only hard work but also consistency, structure, and planning. That's where a personal training plan comes in. Whether you're new to exercise or you're an experienced athlete, having a tailored plan is essential to achieving your goals, staying motivated, and preventing burnout.

In this chapter, we'll guide you through creating your personal training plan for the 7-minute S.I.T. workout. This plan will be designed to suit your needs, goals, and fitness level, ensuring that you stay on track while maximizing your results. By the end of this chapter, you'll be ready to integrate S.I.T. into your routine effectively and with purpose.

1.Setting clear goals

Before diving into any workout plan, it's crucial to define your fitness goals. Understanding what you want to achieve will help shape your workout plan, providing direction and motivation. S.I.T. workouts are incredibly versatile and can be tailored to different goals, whether you want to lose weight, build muscle, increase endurance, or simply improve overall fitness.

A.Goal examples

- **Weight loss:** If your goal is to lose weight, S.I.T. can be an excellent way to burn calories and increase your metabolism. Combining S.I.T. with a healthy, balanced diet will enhance weight loss and fat-burning results.
- **Building strength:** If strength-building is your goal, incorporating more resistance exercises into your S.I.T. routine, such as push-ups, squats, and lunges, can help develop muscle tone and strength.
- **Improving endurance:** If endurance is your focus, you can increase the intensity and duration of your S.I.T. intervals over time to improve cardiovascular health and stamina.
- **Overall fitness:** For general fitness, a mix of different exercises, including bodyweight movements, high-intensity intervals, and strength-building exercises, can help improve your overall health and fitness levels.

Defining your goal will give you clarity and ensure that your training plan stays aligned with your aspirations. Whether it's losing a few pounds or preparing for a race, your goals will guide the structure of your workouts.

2.Understanding your fitness level

Everyone's fitness journey is unique, and it's important to assess your current fitness level before creating a training plan. This self-assessment will help you determine the intensity, duration, and frequency of your workouts, ensuring that you don't push yourself too hard too soon, which could lead to injury or burnout.

A.Assessing your fitness level

- **Beginner:** If you're new to exercise or have been sedentary for a while, it's important to start slowly. Begin with the basic S.I.T. workout, focusing on form and proper technique. Take breaks as needed and gradually increase the intensity as you become more comfortable.
- **Intermediate:** If you're moderately active and have some experience with fitness, you can challenge yourself with more intense intervals and fewer rest periods. Focus on increasing your pace, improving your technique, and targeting more muscle groups.
- **Advanced:** If you're already fit and looking to take your workouts to the next level, increase the duration of your intervals, add variations to your exercises, and even include weights or resistance bands to challenge yourself further.

It's essential to listen to your body and adjust your workouts accordingly. Over time, as your fitness improves, you'll be able to modify your training plan to continue challenging yourself and achieving progress.

3.Building your weekly training plan

A key component of any successful fitness program is consistency. Incorporating the 7-minute S.I.T. workout into your weekly schedule will ensure that you stay on track and make continuous progress toward your goals. Depending on your available time, you can schedule your workouts at different times of the day, ensuring that you remain consistent while balancing work, family, and other commitments.

A.Structuring your week

Here's an example of how to structure your week based on different fitness goals:

- **Weight loss plan:** If you're aiming for weight loss, aim for 4–5 days of S.I.T. per week. You can alternate between full-body workouts and focus on different muscle groups. For example, Monday and Thursday could focus on upper-body exercises, while Tuesday and Friday could focus on lower-body movements. Add a day of active rest, like a light walk or stretching, on Wednesday.
- **Strength plan:** For those focusing on strength, start with 3–4 days of S.I.T. and include exercises such as push-ups, squats, lunges, and planks. Aim to gradually increase the intensity or number of repetitions for these exercises over time.
- **Endurance plan:** If endurance is your goal, aim for 4–6 days of S.I.T. each week. You can increase the length of your work intervals and reduce rest periods as you build cardiovascular strength. One or two days can be active rest, such as light jogging or walking.

The key is to remain consistent with your workouts while incorporating variety to prevent boredom and plateaus. As you progress, continue to adjust your training plan by increasing intensity, adding new exercises, and introducing more challenging variations of the S.I.T. workout.

4.Integrating rest and recovery

While it's tempting to push yourself every day, rest and recovery are vital components of any training plan. Without proper recovery, your body won't have the chance to repair and strengthen the muscles that were worked during the S.I.T. intervals. Additionally, insufficient rest can lead to burnout, fatigue, and increased injury risk.

A.Active rest

On days when you're not doing high-intensity workouts, incorporate active rest. Active rest could include light activities such as walking, stretching, yoga, or foam rolling. This keeps the blood flowing and helps reduce muscle tightness, allowing you to recover and be ready for your next workout session.

B.Full rest days

Full rest days should be incorporated once a week. On these days, avoid any intense exercise. This gives your muscles a chance to recover fully. Full rest days are especially important if you're training at a high intensity, as they allow your body to repair and grow stronger.

5.Tracking your progress

Tracking your progress is essential to staying motivated and ensuring that your training plan is working for you. Regularly measuring your progress helps you identify areas of improvement, see how far you've come, and make necessary adjustments to your training plan.

A.Fitness tracking methods

- **Recording workouts:** Keep a workout journal or use a fitness app to track the exercises, repetitions, sets, and duration of your S.I.T. workouts. Note how you felt during the workout, whether you were able to push harder, or if you struggled with certain exercises.
- **Measuring physical progress:** If weight loss or muscle gain is one of your goals, track your body measurements, weight, and body fat percentage over time. Taking progress pictures can also be a powerful way to see changes in your body composition.
- **Tracking performance:** If your focus is on performance improvement, track your time, intensity, and the number of intervals you complete during each S.I.T. workout. Gradually aim to improve your speed or the number of exercises you complete within the 7-minute window.

6.Adjusting your plan over time

As you get stronger and more accustomed to your S.I.T. workout, you'll need to adapt your training plan to continue challenging your body. Every few weeks, assess how your body feels, whether you're meeting your goals, and if you're ready for more intensity. If you feel that you've plateaued or become bored, consider increasing the duration, frequency, or intensity of your intervals. You can also switch up the exercises to prevent monotony and keep your workouts fresh and exciting.

7.Staying motivated

Creating a personal training plan is about more than just the physical workout—it's about staying motivated and inspired to reach your goals. Here are a few tips to maintain motivation:

- **Set mini goals:** Set weekly or monthly goals to stay focused. These could include completing a certain number of workouts, achieving a specific fitness milestone, or trying a new variation of the S.I.T. workout.
- **Reward yourself:** Celebrate your achievements by treating yourself to a non-food-related reward, such as a new workout outfit or a relaxing day of self-care.
- **Find support:** If you struggle with accountability, consider joining a fitness community or enlisting a workout buddy to keep you motivated.

8.Conclusion

Creating your personal training plan for the 7-minute S.I.T. workout allows you to take control of your fitness journey and tailor your workouts to your individual needs and goals. By setting clear goals, assessing your fitness level, structuring your week, incorporating recovery, tracking progress, and staying motivated, you'll be well on your way to achieving your desired results. Remember, consistency is key, and the most important step is simply getting started.

Ending:

As you conclude your journey through the 7-minute S.I.T. workout plan, remember that success is built on consistency, determination, and an understanding of your own body. By creating a personal training plan tailored to your specific goals and needs, you've laid the foundation for a healthier, stronger, and more confident version of yourself. The beauty of S.I.T. lies in its simplicity and efficiency – just 7 minutes of focused effort can produce significant results, whether you're aiming to lose weight, build strength, increase endurance, or simply improve your overall fitness.

However, the real key to long-term success is integrating your workouts into your daily life and making them a non-negotiable part of your routine. With a clear plan in place, the progress you make will be measurable, and the obstacles you face will feel more manageable. Keep in mind that every small step forward is progress, and every challenge is an opportunity for growth.

As you move forward, remember that fitness is not just about physical transformation – it's about improving your mindset, developing discipline, and gaining confidence in your abilities. Whether you're just starting or have already experienced great results, keep pushing your limits, listening to your body, and embracing the process. By doing so, you'll not only achieve your fitness goals but also create a healthier, more balanced lifestyle that will continue to reward you for years to come.

The journey is yours to take. Stay committed, stay consistent, and above all, enjoy the process. With S.I.T. as part of your fitness routine, you have all the tools you need to succeed. Here's to the next chapter of your journey – one where you keep striving, achieving, and feeling stronger every day.

Made in the USA
Las Vegas, NV
22 May 2025

22493780R00085